RUNNING and WALKING FOR WOMEN OVER 40

RUNNING *and* WALKING FOR WOMEN OVER 40

THE ROAD TO SANITY AND VANITY

KATHRINE SWITZER

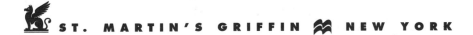 ST. MARTIN'S GRIFFIN ※ NEW YORK

Line illustrations copyright © 1998 by Precision Graphics.

Photos on pgs. 29 and 103 courtesy of FPG International.
Unless otherwise indicated all photos are courtesy of Janeart.

Design by Helene Wald Berinksy

ISBN 0-312-18777-7

First St. Martin's Griffin Edition: May 1998

10   9   8   7   6   5   4

To my mother, Virginia Miller Switzer, and my father, W. Homer Switzer,
who taught me to participate in life, not to spectate,
and to
Arnie Briggs, my first coach,
who showed me how.

CONTENTS

ACKNOWLEDGMENTS

I would like to extend my thanks and gratitude to the many people who helped so much in the writing of this book. First, to my agent, Jennifer Lyons, and my editor, Becky Koh, for their love of sports and their support in this project and in me. Next, to Ellen Kavier whose editing, writing, and research skills made order out of my chaos and without whom completion of the book would have been impossible. My dear friends Jane Kagan Vitiello and Greg Vitiello, who also wrote, listened, advised, and found Ellen. Pamela Cooper, sports historian, writer, and friend, for her valuable contribution. For inspiration and belief, enormous gratitude to publisher and friend Scotty Hart.

To Jim Preston, chairman of Avon Products Inc., for his extraordinary vision, and to Brian Martin and Carolyn Aishton for their faith, as we relaunch Avon Running—Global Women's Circuit.

To my niece and nephew, Anne and Wayne Switzer, for being my sounding boards and telling me what's "in"—and what's not.

To friends and colleagues who eagerly gave expert information, advice, and opinions: Reidun Andersen, Bob Anderson, Gloria Averbuch, Gordon Bakoulis, George Banker, Sharon Barbano, I. W. Barkis,

Ph.D., Ilse Bechthold, Tim Chamberlain, Nancy Clark, Ward Cunningham-Rundles, M.D., J. D. Denton, Barbara Drinkwater, Ph.D., Kaye Durland, Julia Emmons, Jules Esther, Fleet Feet, Inc., Ayne Furman, M.D., Henley Gabeau, Lea Gallardo, Bob Glover, Norm Green, Howard "Jake" Jacobson, Annemarie Jutel, Allen Kagan, M.D., Joyce M. Kim, M.D., Mike Keohane, Zan Knudsen (at last), Judy Mahle Lutter, Arthur Lydiard, Jan McLatchie, Elizabeth Maitland, David Martin, Ph.D., Raleigh Mayer, Joe Miller, M.D., Lorraine Moller, Elizabeth Phillips, Joyce Rankin, Joan Benoit Samuelson, Norb Sander, M.D., Jane Serues, Mona Shangold, M.D., Kathy Smith, Maggie Spilner, Joan Ullyot, Ph.D., Grete Waitz, and Lori Weisenfeld, M.D.

To *Runner's World* magazine, for their evaluation of sports bras.

And last to my family for their unwavering support and especially to my husband, Roger Robinson, Ph.D., whose talent, loyalty, wit, and love never cease to inspire me.

RUNNING *and* WALKING FOR WOMEN OVER 40

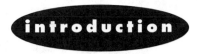

SANITY AND VANITY

As I write this, I've just turned fifty. I was inspired to write this book because at forty-two, or thereabouts, my wonderful and totally pre-dictable body began to change. Suddenly I was encountering gray hair, hot flashes, and mood swings. Running had always provided the ballast in my life, and I turned to it again to help me through these changes. The physical act of running had never failed to correct every imbalance in my life, and I had hope that it would help again. It did! It does! Wonderfully.

When I ran, I didn't feel anxious or depressed. I never had a hot flash on the run; it was as if movement regulated my mood and tem-perature. Best of all, I knew that being out on the road was one of the best things I could be doing possibly to prevent heart disease and osteoporosis—and that made me feel I had some control over my health and my future.

The next eight years were some of the most enlightening of my life, largely made possible by an activity I'd done for twenty-nine years and now find more important than ever. While change is inevitable, running and walking not only enable you to cope with this reality but also offer you a way to triumph over it and feel better than ever.

You're never too old to start. Statistics show that the human body responds positively to fitness at any age. Many active fifty-five-year-old women are in better shape now than they were at twenty-five because of regular exercise. Others are seeking to gain back fitness they lost—and they *can*. I'm counting on my knowledge and my training to build a foundation for a fit and rewarding future. I want to share what I've learned with you, so you can use it, too.

I run or walk every day because it's magic. I'm not kidding. In a funny kind of way, running has given me everything I have or am.

Running and walking keep me sane. In the purest sense, it is a little window of time on my own, or with friends, when I can be free of everything else. With this freedom, I can create, dream, or just drift along and enjoy nature around me. It's my space. My sacred alone, peaceful time, and nobody can invade it. In a world full of chaos, pressure, unpredictability, and constant demands, where everybody seems to want a piece of me, that hour a day gives me a chance for a quiet perspective, and it allows me to control much of my destiny. I have found that if I can control my body and give a little peace to my soul, I can transfer that power into all other aspects of my life.

And, to top everything, running or walking is so simple. It's wonderful how something so simple can give so much back to you, and that may be another element of it's magic.

Ever since I began running when I was thirteen, there was a palpable difference between the days I ran and those I didn't: My running days had more significance. Missing a day wasn't a major tragedy or anything—sometimes you can't help it or just don't feel like it. A day I didn't run was just a day without a bonus, a bonus that enriched my life in so many ways.

My daily outing these days may be a walk, a slow jog, or a run—it has manifested itself over the years in various forms. After early years of discovery and struggle to cocky years of invincibility, I moved into the arduous and pressure-filled years of world-class competition and training.

In my thirties, I gave up serious competitive running for a career that had room for only the barest minimum of fitness running. In my forties, however, when I had my own business and more flexibility, I decided to treat myself to more consistency in my daily running. I not only found renewed fitness but also discovered differences and changes in my body. Now, at fifty, I am poised for the next level.

In all of these eras of running and walking, training hard or easy, doing less or more, the activity has never failed to keep me fit, energetic, positive, and the same weight I was when I was sixteen years old. In fact, running has never failed to give me back more than I put into it. There is not much in life that offers that kind of return.

Despite thirty-seven years of experience, I can still remember the difficulty of starting and the struggle to progress. I can remember what it was like to feel jiggly and conspicuous. I learned fast the single hardest part about exercise: getting out the door! And I created techniques for eliminating excuses. Later, I learned how to stay fit on twenty minutes of running a day in the midst of career pressures and traveling around the world. Through running, I learned marvelous lessons in success, failure, humility, and mortality that have served me well in business and life. And maybe most important, I learned how not to feel guilty or defeated when I missed days, turning them around so I was more motivated and better focused the next time I ran.

I have learned that somewhere after forty, your body begins to change. At twenty-five, I would have told you that I'd always be strong and lithe; at fifty, it's astonishing how closely I've succeeded, but I still have changed. My body wants to age—veins want to show, cellulite is harder to take off, my skin is looser. Although I am determined to stall that process as much as possible, I now have to deal with the fact that my body gets niggles and twinges that it never had before and just doesn't snap back as fast as it did.

But the point is this: It still snaps back! So, although I can't control everything, I can still control a lot. For women who are only beginning fitness programs at forty, fifty, or beyond, this response is nothing short of dramatic. Many find that, for the first time ,they can reach the weight they want to be and get into better physical condition. Women over forty who have been reasonably active all their lives can find a new outlet for their energy in age-group sports events—some easily outrace people young enough to be their children!

Every day I'm finding more ways to be fit, trim, healthy, energetic, and positive while dealing with my changing body. I have plenty of room for improvement, and my challenge at fifty is to find ways to keep fit that require no more than the hour a day I'm willing to give. Anybody can look great if she has plenty of money and is willing to work out several hours a day. But most of us have to live in the real world, where that's not possible. This book gives you the tools to achieve fitness without spending time and money you don't have.

But to get results, you need to get started—that's your most important commitment. Twenty minutes of exercise a day, every day, will get you on the road to sanity, where you feel in control of your life. Thirty minutes a day, every day, will get you on the road to vanity, where you can control your weight, restore skin and muscle tone, and feel great about your body.

Before you say "I just don't have time," remember that the time doesn't have to be all at once. Fifteen minutes in the morning and fifteen minutes at noon or after work give you the thirty minutes you need. Before you think of a second excuse, remember that we always have time to do the things we really want or that are truly important. Your health, your fitness, your sanity (and, yes, even your vanity) are priorities. If you don't feel good about yourself, you can't feel good about much else.

For much of my life, I've been a pioneer: As one of the first woman marathoners, I achieved fame first by registering for and wearing a starting number in the 1967 Boston Marathon, which banned women runners. By running in that race, I debunked the idea that a woman couldn't thrive and succeed running long distances.

To prove that my physical capability was not unique, I then spent the next ten years organizing women's races in more than twenty-five countries as part of the Avon running series. The races demonstrated that women everywhere not only wanted to run and walk, but that they *could.* These pioneering events laid the trail for millions more women, and they resulted in a small social revolution: Women everywhere, regardless of age, size, or capability, began to experience the same joy, magic, and accomplishment that I had discovered as a young woman. With this demonstrated interest among women around the world, I worked with other women to lobby the International Olympic Committee to include a women's marathon in the Olympic Games. We were successful! The women's marathon became an official event beginning in the 1984 Los Angeles Olympic Games, creating a huge goal for women with talent and an inspiration for us all.

In those early years, I was the only woman I knew who ran. There were no women's gyms, no walking groups, no guidelines, no women's shoes, shorts, or bras. Every time I ran longer, people tried to convince me that the earth was flat—any day I'd fall off the edge and suffer dire consequences like big legs, a mustache, or a "displaced" uterus, all dreadful, made-up myths. We know now how ignorant that kind of thinking is, but we also know how much we are held back by these myths and our own fears.

Now I find I am a pioneer again, but I am no longer alone: There are many thousands of you over age forty who also are ready to challenge myth and tradition. Like me, you are determined that aging and the changes it brings will not deprive you of fitness, energy, and good looks. At the same time, the physical and mental shifts occurring after age forty pose challenges. Once again, we are charting our own map.

Those who missed the fitness movement as young adults should take heart: Your happiest and fittest days can still be ahead of you. Those of us lucky enough to have caught the train to fitness as young adults are experiencing a midlife that our parents and grandparents never dreamed possible. But until now, we've had no guidelines. Now we have this book, and we have each other. Let's go forward together as pioneers of the next generation of fitness, pushing back the barriers and limitations of age, just as we did the myths and ignorance surrounding women athletes in the past.

Have fun. Be fearless. Be free.

Golden Rules for Running and Walking

1. Make running or walking a priority in your daily schedule. It is an investment in yourself; it's not selfish or indulgent.

2. Running or walking regularly makes you feel good about yourself. And when you feel good about yourself, your relationships with others are better, as well.

3. Try to run or walk every day, until it becomes a part of your regular routine. Then, if you wind up doing it only three times a week, you're still maintaining your fitness level.

4. Running or walking is the single most time-efficient method of fitness. If you invest thirty minutes a day in your workout, you get back thirty minutes of benefits, plus a lot more.

5. If you can't find a full thirty minutes to do your entire walk or run, try doing fifteen minutes in the morning and fifteen minutes in the evening.

6. Something is always better than nothing. Even ten minutes can give you a sense of accomplishment and contribute to your fitness.

7. Don't feel guilty about missing a workout. Just start again when you can.

8. Invest in a good pair of walking shoes for walking and running shoes for running. Tennis shoes won't do. Buy your shoes at an athletic store where the salespeople are runners or walkers.

9. Find a training partner. It's motivating when someone's waiting for you, particularly when it's dark, cold, or rainy. It's also a good safety precaution.

10. Move fast enough to puff a little and work up a sweat but avoid going too fast too soon. Your goal is sustained exercise that is comfortable but keeps you working. If you can't carry on a conversation while you're running or walking, you're going too fast.

11. Put ice on sore muscles for about ten minutes after a workout. This speeds recovery.

12. Walk or run with your kids, spouse, the dog. It's a great way to combine family time with exercise.

13. Drink water all day long. No matter how much you think you're drinking, it's almost never as much as you need.

14. Diets don't work, because they slow metabolism. Only exercise truly keeps fat off because it raises metabolism. Eat a well-balanced diet that is lower in fat and higher in carbohydrates; you'll have the energy to exercise harder and burn even more calories!

15. Keep a training log. You'll be amazed and proud of your progress (You also won't skip workouts!)

16. Leave your Walkman at home or in the gym. You need all your senses alert when you're running or walking outdoors.

17. Have a goal. Whether it's completing your first mile or entering a local fun run six months from now, a goal keeps you motivated.

chapter 1

GETTING OUT THE DOOR

There is an expression among even the most advanced runners that getting your shoes on is the hardest part of any workout. If you've been finding it hard to start running or walking, don't feel alone. Every athlete faces this problem at one time or another.

Don't put off starting to run or walk anymore. Embrace it. Make it a priority. The best way to start is to choose a date on your calendar: Running/Walking Day! Get psyched. Prepare for it. Call some friends and say, "Let's go for a walk [or run] on Tuesday!"

Maybe you just want to do this quietly for yourself. Either way, you've just set your first goal. You

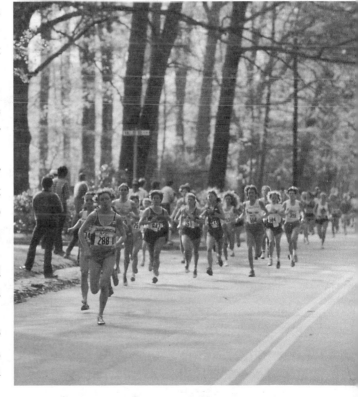

didn't think it would be this easy, did you? Well, it is and it isn't. Following are some things you should do before you literally step out the door for your first run or walk.

Making a commitment to exercise, getting a preexercise physical, determining your level of fitness, and setting a goal helps ensure that you've chosen the right path for yourself and that you are starting at the proper level. There are also tips on such fundamentals as breathing, cooldowns, warm-ups, stretching, and measuring your aerobic capacity.

Think of this information as the foundation for your workout. Once you've built it, then it's time to start running or walking.

Make a Commitment to Running or Walking

No matter what your ultimate running or walking goal is, you first have to decide that you want to make exercise a part of your life. When you've done that, everything else follows naturally. You'll find time for running and walking in your busy schedule. Family and friends will respect your undertaking and not interfere with your decision.

In a larger sense, making this commitment means you've opened a door to a more proactive and self-reliant lifestyle. Your workout is just one step. It can give you the power to reshape other areas of your life as well.

Get a Physical Before You Start

Your body goes through a tremendous number of changes after forty. Adding exercise to the mix, particularly if you've never done it before or haven't done it for a long time, increases that burden. Before starting to run or walk, have a physical exam and tell your doctor you are planning an exercise program. Even though running or walking is probably one of the best things you can do for yourself at this time, you may have some pre-existing medical problems that need monitoring if you exercise. The same thing is true if you are on special medications.

When you are forty-five, fifty-five, or sixty-five, your bones and muscles are very different from those you had at twenty-five, so your doctor may recommend some testing before you start an exercise program. For example, if you are in menopause, the doctor may suggest a bone scan to determine your bone density, which will measure your vulnerability to osteoporosis. Your doctor may discover that you have muscle or bone weaknesses and recommend that you begin your exercise program more modestly—walking for several months before considering running. The doctor may also recommend stretching or strength-building exercises that will prevent injury when you start to exercise. He or she may also suggest that you alternate running or walking with swimming and stretching, for instance, as the new sensation of pounding on a hard surface might be too much in the beginning of your training for uninitiated joints, bones, and muscles.

A preexercise checkup is also a very good baseline indicator. You can start measuring real physical improvement from this time. It's also helpful to have a doctor who shares your desire for self-improvement. If you are getting a less than enthusiastic response from your doctor about your exercise plans when there is no real physical reason for his or her objection, it might be the right time to consider seeing a different doctor.

There is another important reason for having a checkup. Beginning to run or walk signifies a change in attitude toward your health and well-being and who controls it. Starting now, *you* are taking charge of your physical well-being. Most women age forty and over traditionally took a passive role when it came to questions of health. They learned just to obey doctor's orders without questioning them or feeling they had the right to be a part of the decision-making process regarding their health. This visit to the doctor could change that old relationship forever.

The good news is that no matter how old you are, the body is always regenerating itself. Since exercise makes every organ, muscle, and bone better and stronger, every day you exercise is an opportunity to improve your body as it re-creates itself!

A personal note:

I've known some women who constantly complained about being tired but wanted to begin a fitness program. As a result of their preexercise physical they found out that they had been anemic for years. By taking iron supplements and changing their diet, they started down the path of complete fitness—inside and out. Others use this time to make sure they include an annual mammogram in their exam.

Determine Your Level of Fitness

What shape are you in? Perhaps you are what's known as a weekend warrior—a woman who plays sports on the weekend but never at any other time. Or you don't participate in organized sports, but you are a wife, mother, and worker, so you're constantly active and on the move. In order to more accurately determine your fitness level, consult the following lists. They provide measurement tools to help you evaluate your fitness level. If you see yourself on both lists—you smoke but are not overweight—go with the list that best reflects your overall level of activity. If you are still unsure about your fitness level, start at the earliest stage of the program. You can always move ahead if you're able to handle that level comfortably and need a greater challenge.

You're a *real beginner* if:

- You smoke.
- You just quit smoking.
- You've never done any systematic exercise.
- You haven't exercised systematically for ten years.
- You're more than twenty pounds overweight.

- You commute to work and have a desk job.
- You get tired shopping.

You're an *intermediate beginner* and in better shape than you think if:

- You walk to work.
- You are not overweight.
- You've never smoked, or you quit at least five years ago.
- You are constantly moving on the job, even if it is technically a desk job.
- You do outdoor things, including gardening.
- You can be on your legs shopping for two hours and not think about it.
- You choose to walk instead of driving to do errands if you can accomplish your chores in the same amount of time.

You're an *advanced or above beginner* if:

- You play sports or do other fitness activities, such as tennis, golf, swimming or aerobics, fairly regularly.
- You spend a lot of time on your feet each day moving around.
- You choose active vacations that involve sports like hiking, skiing, and bicycling
- Besides being quite active, you read a lot about women's health, fitness, and sports.

Set a Goal and Write It Down

Establishing a goal gives focus and commitment to your efforts. Putting the goal on paper gives it a significance beyond those easily set—and just as easily broken—New Year's resolutions we all make.

At the same time, don't hesitate to alter your goal if circumstances change. Perhaps a new job or family responsibilities make it impossible to keep your original goal. Instead of abandoning it completely, simply make the necessary adjustment.

Be realistic about your goal. Make it high enough to push yourself but not so ambitious that it can't be reasonably attained. If you start with a modest goal, when you reach it you can set another, higher one, to strive for. Pretty soon you'll have a record of accomplishments—and that will feel great.

If you're unsure about how to set an objective, here are some worthwhile goals for different levels of fitness:

- To walk or run three times a week for twelve consecutive weeks.
- To walk or run three to four times a week until you can easily complete a 5K distance (3.1 mile) and enter a local fun run, race or fitness walk.
- To gradually replace smoking with exercise by cutting out a cigarette a day and replacing it with a brisk walk and deep breathing.
- To lose half of your *excess* weight over the next year by running or walking three times a week and maintaining your fitness program.
- To follow a program and be able to walk or run a 10K race (6.2 miles) in six months.
- To compete in your age group in an upcoming race or meet.
- In addition to your regular running or walking program, to incorporate extra physical activity in your normal day. For instance, take the stairs instead of an elevator, walk rather than drive to do local errands, walk or bike with your family or friends rather than going to the movies. Write these changes down in your running or walking log.
- To become a thirty-minutes-a-day runner or walker.
- To become a forty-five-minutes-a-day runner or walker.
- To complete a marathon.

Have fun with your goals. Dream of what you can be and where you want to go and then use your goals to take you there. And don't forget to congratulate yourself when you reach a goal. Let everyone know—share the glory and accomplishment. Besides feeling good about yourself, you may inspire someone else.

TIP

It's easier to replace one habit with another rather than to give up something. When you give up something without replacing it, you feel deprived and resentful, even when it's a bad habit. Running or walking temporarily suppresses the appetite and raises your mood, just as smoking does for some people , so it works well as a replacement activity. Soon it will be a new habit.

Keep a Running or Walking Log

Write down your running or walking schedule, then record the exercise you have done each day. You can buy a fancy log from a bookstore for this purpose or use a school composition notebook, a desk diary, or a calendar posted on your refrigerator. Keep notes on how you felt during your workout, what you saw, or any things you want to add to your routine. Check your actual workouts against your goal to see how you are progressing. Writing notes gives you a concrete assessment of how much you are actually doing. If you don't write it down, it is very easy to fool yourself into thinking that you are doing more than you really are. By the same token, you may be surprised by how much you've accomplished.

Running and Walking: How Do I Breathe?

Every beginner asks this question, and after a week of walking or running, she never thinks about it again. The best advice is not to *think* too much about how to breathe, just walk or run and let it happen naturally!

Here are some hints to help you breathe more easily.

- Breathe through both your nose and mouth. You need all the air you can get. Air is 80 percent oxygen, and oxygen energizes you.

- Don't try to breathe in rhythm with your steps, or on a count, or by concentrating on taking deep breaths. Breathing has a mind and rhythm of its own; let it seek its own level.

- You shouldn't feel totally out of breath when you run. If you do, it's usually a sign that you need to adjust your workout. Perhaps you're running too fast or talking too much. Maybe you're too excited or anxious about something. Or maybe you are just going uphill. If you become winded, slow down or stop until your get your breath back. Then start again, this time at a more moderate pace.

- Getting *somewhat* breathless is sometimes an important part of training. You need to push slightly to expand your lungs and develop more breathing capacity. When you move faster and feel breathlessness coming on, back off a little and slow down without stopping. When you catch your breath again, you can start to pick up your pace. The combination of pushing and then relaxing is excellent training. Soon you will go faster and farther. There even will be periods of time when you'll feel you can run forever and never be breathless.

- Don't worry about taking air in—think about getting stale air out. A forced, hard exhale with your hads over your head several times during a workout always feels refreshing. It also relieves side aches, called stitches.

- If you're running in cold weather, breathe slowly through your nose. When you start running in subzero temperatures, hold a scarf or gloved hand over your mouth and nose to slightly warm the air first. This will prevent you from "gulping" freezing air. Gradually, as you run faster and warm up your body, your nose and mouth will get accustomed to the cold. Before you are able to do fast and breathless running comfortably in very cold air, you need to train for a while in those conditions. (There are more cold weather training tips in Chapter 6.)

- Is there really a "second wind"? It seems like magic, but it's a normal occurrence. Just when you are walking or running along and feeling utterly breathless, you suddenly begin to feel better and can breathe normally. There is nothing mysterious about it. What's happened is that you have slowed down very slightly so that you are getting enough air again. The difference between easy and not so easy running is often imperceptible to a beginner. This happens to elite racers, too, who get a second wind when they adjust their pace and get their body warmed up to accommodate the work load. You can get your own second wind by simply slowing a bit. It feels a lot better than having to stop.

- If you really feel you're having trouble breathing through your nose, ask your doctor to check the inside of your nose for obstructions, such as a deviated septum or polyps. This kind of problem can be corrected, and you'll feel much more comfortable while running.

Priming the Pump: The Warm-Up

The purpose of the warm-up is to start blood circulating and prepare muscles for the work ahead. It may also help in preventing injuries because cold, tight muscles are not ready to respond to new work. A good warm-up also makes the workout a lot more comfortable because running or walking on tight muscles can be uncomfortable. It's especially important if you exercise early in the morning, when muscles are tightest.

The more intensive the performance, the longer and more thorough the warm-up should be. Elite athletes spend an hour or more warming up for an event that may last ten seconds! But for you, the warm-up should take only a few minutes and can be mostly incorporated as part of the walk or run itself.

BASIC WARM-UP: Start walking; swing your arms in gentle windmills; shrug your shoulders and roll your head. Stop and bend from side to side, gently bend over and hang from the waist; straighten up slowly, and walk again, very slowly at first, gradually building your speed until you're into your regular workout.

Towel-Off: The Cooldown

At the end of your running workout, slow down and begin walking; at the end of your walking workout, slow down and start to amble. Easy exercise helps remove lactic acid that has built up in your muscles from your harder work—lactic acid causes soreness. Walk until you've completely caught your breath, swinging your arms, etc., as you did in the warm-up.

Then, slowly and gently perform the stretching exercises that follow. Don't overstretch; just try to achieve the feeling you are smoothing out the kinks. Stretching after your workout rather than before, is often more productive, since your muscles are now warm and flexible.

You want to stretch warm muscles, so if it is cold outside, do your stretching indoors before you get cold. If it is hot outside and air conditioned indoors, stay outside to stretch. In either case, if you get chilled, take a warm shower before stretching.

A Basic Stretching Routine

The following stretches work for all of the running and walking programs described in this chapter. You can use them to stretch your muscles and provide a relaxed cooldown after you run.

Calf

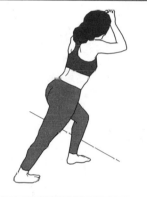

Lean against a tree, pole, or wall with your forearms, your head resting on your hands. Bend one leg and place it on the ground in front of you, with the other leg straight behind. Slowly move your hips forward, keeping your lower back flat. Keep the heel of the straight leg on the ground, toes pointed straight. Hold for forty seconds for each leg

---

Calf and Achilles tendon

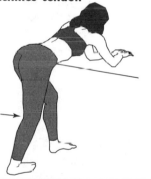

Hold onto a flat surface and lower your hips, bending your back leg slightly at the knee. The toes of your back leg should be pointed straight or slightly toe-in. The front leg is bent. Hold stretch for fifteen seconds for each leg.

Lower back, hips, groin, and hamstring

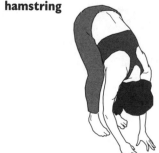

Stand with feet shoulder width apart and pointed straight ahead. Slowly bend forward from the hips. Keep knees slightly bent during the stretch to ease the stress on your back. Relax your neck and arms and let your arms hang down. Bend to the point where you feel a slight stretch in the back of your legs. Hold for thirty seconds.

Knees, shins, back, ankles, Achilles tendon, and deep groin

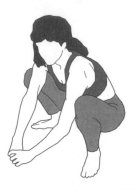

Squat, from a standing position, with your feet flat and toes pointed slightly outward. Heels should be 4–12" apart, depending on how flexible you are and how accustomed to the stretch. Keep you knees straight over your big toes. Hold for twenty seconds. May be difficult at first.

Repeat stretch for lower back, hips, groin, and hamstrings

Hold for thirty seconds.

Ankles

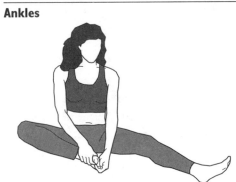

Sit with one leg out to the side, knee slightly bent. Take the other foot in both hands and rotate your ankle clockwise and counterclockwise with a slight resistance from your hand. Repeat fifteen times in each direction for both feet.

Quadriceps

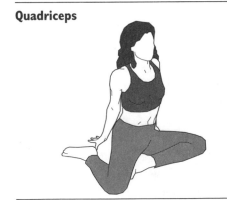

Sit with your right leg bent and your right heel just outside of your right hip. Bend your left leg and place the sole of your left foot next to the inside of your upper right leg. Place your hands on the floor behind you to support your upper body. Hold for thirty seconds for each leg.

Hamstrings

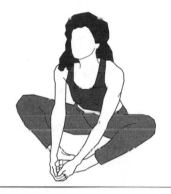

Straighten your right leg with the knee slightly bent; move the sole of your left foot until it is just touching the inside of your right thigh. Slowly bend forward from your hips to create the feeling of an easy stretch in the hamstrings. Hold for thirty seconds for each leg. Bend forward from your hips, not by bending your head over your leg.

Groin

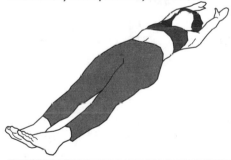

Sitting on the ground, put the soles of your feet together and hold onto your toes. Gently pull yourself forward, bending from the hips, until you gently stretch the groin. Hold for forty seconds. Create the stretch by pushing forward from your hips, not by rounding your head and shoulders.

Rib cage, abdominals, spine, shoulders, arms, ankles, and feet

Lie on the ground with your lower back flat and your arms stretched out above your head. Stretch both your arms and legs at the same time. Hold for five seconds and repeat three times.

Groin

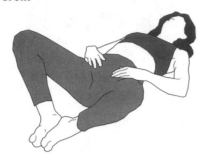

Lie on your back, knees bent and soles of your feet together. Hold for sixty seconds.

Lower back and hips

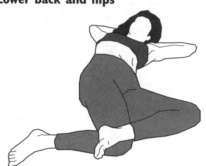

Lying on the ground, bring your knees together and place your feet on the floor. Lift your left leg over your right knee and use your left leg to pull your right leg toward the ground. Keep your upper back, head, and shoulders flat on the ground. Hold for twenty-five seconds for each side.

Gaining and Measuring Your Aerobic Benefit

Once you become a thirty-minute runner or walker, you've entered the area where you can begin to reap the cardiovascular benefits of aerobic exercise. An aerobic exercise is any moderately intensive activity—such as running, biking and walking—that raises your heart rate and can be sustained for more than two minutes. You start getting aerobic benefits if you walk at your target heart rate for a minimum of twenty minutes three times a week.

To gain a good, safe aerobic benefit from your workout, you need to exercise hard enough for your heart to beat at its target rate, which is 60 to 80 percent of your maximum heart rate.

There is an easy way to discover both your maximum and target heart rates. Your maximum heart rate is determined by subtracting your age from 220. Your target heart rate is a zone 60 to 80 percent of that number. If you are an average fifty-year-old, your maximum heart rate is 170 (220–50). Your target heart rate is 102 to 136 beats per minute.

When you exercise within this range, you improve your heart and vascular system, and you burn fat. You will also notice that your resting heart rate becomes slower, another measure of your improved conditioning.

Check your heart rate during your walk or run to see if you're working within your target heart rate zone. Press the first two fingers of one hand *gently* against the opposite inner wrist just under your thumb, until you find the pulse or on your carotid artery just under the angle of your jaw. Keep moving while you take your pulse. Count the beats for ten seconds and then multiply that number by six. To check on your conditioning, take your resting pulse when you start your program and then occasionally later on. Do it when you first wake up in the morning, while you're still in bed.

chapter 2

STARTING HERE, STARTING NOW

THE BEGINNING FOR RUNNERS AND WALKERS

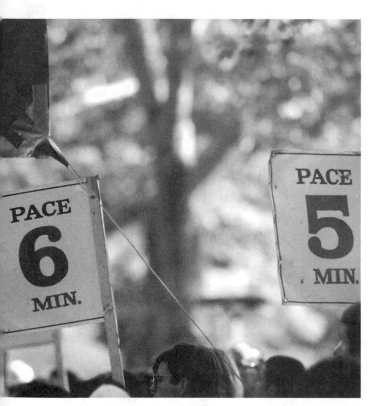

All women must walk before they can run.

Whether you're out for your very first run or your returning to the road after several years away, or if you intend to become a regular walker, you should begin by putting on a watch, going outside, and walking purposefully for a few minutes. For some of you, this might be five minutes; for others, fifteen. Don't push, don't hurt, and don't get breathless. Have fun! Walking and running should always be fun, even when you increase your physical challenges later in your program.

For the next three weeks, continue going out for a walk. Try to go every other day, with a minimum of three times a week. Each time you walk, add a minute to your walk and try to go just a bit faster.

TIP

If you miss a workout, don't feel guilty. Just start again as soon as possible. If you miss a lot of days, you may need to start again very gradually, but don't fret. The important thing is doing it!

By the second or third week, some intermediate walking beginners may start to feel a bit restless and want to move on.

Beginning walkers will want to remain at this phase for as long as it takes to feel comfortable. A good guideline is to increase your distance or time in the activity by 10 percent a week. When you're ready to start your fitness walking program, turn to chapter 4.

Those who want to run will notice that at times during their walks they break into slow runs or jogs. This is a good time to experiment with very easy running. As you walk, pick out a mailbox or telephone pole fifty to sixty yards away and very gently break into a slow run and jog to it. Walk again to catch your breath and repeat this process in all your walks, adding more and longer running phases. You're now ready for your first real running program.

Real running beginners may take weeks or even several months before they can reach this stage, depending on their original physical condition. This is usually the crossroads where a true beginner determines whether she will stay a walker or wants to move on to become a runner.

A personal note:

Some people need to run in the morning to start the day; other people need to run in the evening to get over the day. I am definitely in the latter category—the evening run ends my day just as assuredly as a drink ends many other people's. It is a time for me to get out the frazzles, kick some butt, sort out the emotions of the day, and prepare for the next. Inevitably, I come back refreshed, civilized, and ready for a happy evening. Plenty of my friends run in the morning and say it sets them up for a perfect day. To each her own. I find just getting out of bed in the morning a big challenge!

Running: Form and Fundamentals.

How do you run? The answer seems obvious: You put one foot in front of the other. Right? Yet it is one of the most frequently asked questions because running is not quite *that* easy. There are a few rules to follow.

First, you have to move from walking to running. How do you get started? Try this method. Go outside and start walking. Walk a bit faster. Then pick up the pace some more and sort of shuffle along; you're moving as quickly as you were in the first walk, but it's actually easier. Shuffle just a bit faster, landing on your heels and rolling forward. Now you're jogging, but it should feel just as easy as fast walking.

RUNNING FORM. Run with your shoulders back and your arms and hands relaxed. Bend your elbows at your waist with the palms of your hands facing each other, as if you were getting ready to put your hand in your pant's pockets. Keep your hands loosely cupped.

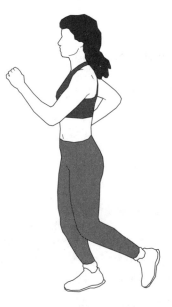

Let your arms swing naturally, forward and back, parallel to each other. Don't let your arms cross in front of your body, because this tends to twist your body.

As you run, try to swing your legs out in front of you, following your arms. Keep feet and knees facing forward.

Keep your head erect and your eyes focused about ten to fifteen yards in front of you. Don't look straight down at your feet. Your chin should be parallel to the ground. Keeping your head up helps your form and allows you to see more of the scenery. It also allows you to see any obstacle that is in your path before it's too late.

Nobody wants to say she's jogging; everyone wants to say she's running. Right now, you probably feel foolish calling this action running, but in time, when you start jogging longer and longer, you'll be calling yourself a runner. And you'll be right!

A personal note:

I began running as a young girl with the very method described here. I thought I would never get beyond the one-mile mark, and then later, the three-mile mark. My body would progress, and then it would just seem to hit a plateau, and it was a while before I could get it to progress again. Eventually, I became a marathon (26.2 miles) runner, and the plateau effect began again as I started a program of getting faster. Some elite runners work very hard for a year or two before they suddenly make a breakthrough.

chapter 3

A RUNNING PROGRAM

MAKING STRIDES FOR SANITY AND VANITY

Walkers: Go to Chapter 4, "A Walking Program."

Runners: Start here.

After you have done the beginning walking and running program for a few weeks, and are comfortable with your workouts, you may be ready to take the next step. The following schedule is designed to turn you into a continuous thirty-minute runner in ten weeks. Try to run three or four days a week. On the days you don't run, either rest or do some other training—biking, swimming, or weight training—to give your body time to recuperate from running.

Not everyone can complete this program in ten weeks. If you need more time, take it. You're on your own schedule, and nobody is judging you!

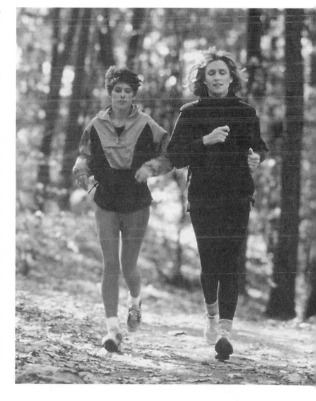

HOW TO BECOME A 30-MINUTE RUNNER IN 10 WEEKS

WEEK 1: Walk 30 minutes a day, at least three times a week.

WEEK 2: Continue week-one workout but pick up the pace, pump your arms. Break a sweat!

WEEK 3: Walk 8 minutes. Run 2 minutes. Walk 1 minute (repeat this 3-minute session 5 times). Walk 8 minutes.

WEEK 4: Walk 6 minutes, run 4 minutes. Repeat three times.

WEEK 5: Walk 5 minutes, run 5 minutes. Repeat three times.

WEEK 6: Walk 3 minutes, run 7 minutes. Repeat three times.

WEEK 7: Walk 2 minutes, run 8 minutes. Repeat three times.

WEEK 8: Walk 1 minute, run 9 minutes. Repeat three times.

WEEK 9: Walk 1 minute, run 14 minutes. Repeat twice.

WEEK 10: Run 30 minutes.

TIP

You should always be able to carry on a conversation while you're running. If you can't, you're going too fast.

A personal note:

I can't stress enough the need for you to make a commitment to a routine, even though I also believe that you shouldn't feel guilty about missing a workout. If you know that you usually run on Tuesday, Saturday, and Sunday, you focus on those days. Putting off your running for a day or two can start a pattern of procrastination. You miss days, mess up your schedule, and become discouraged. If it's on the calendar, you'll do it. Even when you think you're tired, doing your run energizes you!

Getting Longer, Getting Stronger: Becoming a One-Hour Runner

Becoming a thirty-minute runner may be your ultimate goal, or you may want to revise your goal and crank it up a notch or two.

One of the best new goals for the thirty-minute runner is to try to run for a longer time. Not only is it easily measurable but it also gives a tremendous sense of satisfaction. Once you've finished a longer run, it's a real kick to drive over the same roads and see how much distance you covered on foot. You'll feel a sense of ownership over the territory you've run.

Treadmill runners don't experience this same kind of claim to territory. However, you can get a similar sense by seeing the treadmill odometer register more mileage, or by watching the clock and seeing your staying power grow from workout to workout.

Even if you think you plan to be a thirty-minute runner every day and leave it at that, give some thought to increasing your distance for the following reasons:

- Being able to run for forty-five minutes or even an hour gives a tremendous sense of confidence and power. If you feel good doing thirty minutes, you'll feel a hundred times better doing an hour!

- Being able to run longer is a safety factor; if you get lost, you can keep going longer.

- Thirty minutes a day raises metabolism and begins a process of gradual weight reduction. But when you run for an hour or more, you get into real fat-burning territory. That is one reason why a long run once a week is so critical to many serious training schedules and is an important component of a good weight-loss program.

- Once you have safely and gradually worked up to it, being able to run for an hour is a good means of creating leg strength. When you have strong legs, you can work more easily on getting faster.

A personal note:

Running is incredibly addictive—not only because it feels good, but when you accomplish a distance, you are often instinctively challenged to try to go farther. Many women have never attempted this kind of physical test before. Once you know you can do it, you become curious about how much more you can do and thrilled by the excitement of trying.

Becoming a One-Hour Runner

The key component of this program is the one long run per week. It builds up endurance and lays the foundation for further progress.

WEEKS 1–3: Right now you are running 30 minutes a day, three days a week. Your weekly commitment of time is 90 minutes. Continue this for three weeks.

WEEK 4: Run 30 minutes, 29 minutes, 35 minutes. Weekly total: 94 minutes.

WEEK 5: Run 30 minutes, 32 minutes, 38 minutes. Weekly total: 100 minutes.

WEEK 6: Run 30 minutes, 33 minutes, 41 minutes. Weekly total: 104 minutes.

WEEK 7: Run 30 minutes, 34 minutes, 45 minutes. Weekly total: 109 minutes.

WEEK 8: Run 30 minutes, 36 minutes, 49 minutes. Weekly total: 115 minutes.

WEEK 9: Run 30 minutes, 38 minutes, 54 minutes. Weekly total: 122 minutes.

WEEK 10: Run 30 minutes, 40 minutes, 60 minutes. Weekly total: 130 minutes.

When you are trying to increase your distance, some days feel good and others feel awful. Listen to your body. Be willing to back off. There is no hurry. These schedules are designed for the best possible circumstances, and sometimes you just need more time to adapt. Never move on to the next higher distance until you feel totally comfortable with the one you did today. I can remember once doing the same mileage for three weeks before I felt I had the strength to add a bit more.

Running Tips for Increasing Time and Mileage

- Running every other day is important in the early stages because it allows for recovery. Progress is made only when you push yourself a bit farther, but to make a gain you have to recover from it. This principle is known to all athletes as "hard-easy" training.

- You may want to start running more than three times a week to break up your total minutes into more manageable segments. For instance, in week 8, you may have two days available for twenty-minute runs, but not a solid thirty-eight minutes. That's okay. In this program, there are only two important components: total weekly time and a weekly continuous long run.

- After your long run of the week, *always* take a day off from running.

- Even if you normally run alone, finding a partner during this building-up stage can be a big help because there will be times when you can use some moral support. It's also nice to have a partner for the long run because it makes the time go faster. Doing longer runs with a partner adds to your safety. You may be going farther than ever before and you can't be a hundred percent sure of how you'll react or how tired you'll get, so it's nice to have someone with you.

- If at any time you feel like walking during a run, *do it*. If you were swimming, you'd sink, but in running many people walk to catch their breath or ease a side cramp, or because they are suddenly very hot. Brief walks are not cheating, nor are they a sign you are a wimp. On the contrary, a few minutes of walking can be a pause that refreshes or a moment of time that restores your energy for the rest of the run. From that point of view, walking can be a valuable training aid.

A personal note:

Sometimes I find myself walking for a few seconds or even a minute during a workout without quite realizing why. I've ceased to worry about this; it seems to have to do with getting my body into a better rhythm or adjusting to heat or perhaps an early too-fast pace. And going uphill! I often walk part of a hill, especially when I can see that walking it is just as fast as running it!

Converting Time to Mileage

I take the approach that running for time is more important than running for mileage since our lives today are so dominated by time. The easiest way to find out how far you are going is to run on a local high school or college track. These tracks are a standard 400 meters (440 yards), and four laps equal one mile. A few bike paths and nature trails have mileage markers on them, or you can check your mileage on a car odometer. However, car odometers often indicate that the route is longer than it really is. This is one area where treadmill runners have an advantage. The odometers on their machines really work.

It's nice to know how far you actually are going, if for no other reason than to brag about it! Also, if you decide to enter a race or fun run you'll need to have some idea of how long it will take you to cover the distance. Most of these runs are 5-kilometer (also called 5K, which is

3.1 miles) or 10-kilometer (10K, which is 6.2 miles) events. It sounds like a lot, but you'll be pleasantly surprised to find that you are probably capable of covering these distances by this point in your training without having to walk.

If you want to get a fairly accurate idea of how far you run, do the following: Go to your local high school or college track and time yourself with a stopwatch as you run one mile (four laps) at your regular training pace. How long did this take you? If it took you ten minutes, for example, you run at a ten-minute-per-mile pace. So if you run thirty minutes a day, you run three miles a day. If you run a total of 120 minutes a week, you can assume that your weekly mileage is about twelve miles. Therefore, you can easily calculate how much more you need to do to be ready for a fun run or race. A schedule follows, using mileage instead of time.

TIP

Real runners talk about their mileage in terms of weekly, not daily, mileage. The novice always asks you, "How many miles a day do you run?" and the regular runner always has to stop to figure it out. Almost all runners train on some version of the "hard-easy" principle, rarely doing the same number of miles or time every day. So when runners talk to each other, they know that it's the week's accumulated mileage that counts. Be cool—quote your weekly mileage!

Getting Ready for a Fun Run or Race

A good rule if you want to enter a race and you're not sure you can do the mileage is to triple the distance of the race and make sure your total *weekly* mileage exceeds it. For instance, if the race is 3.1 miles, you should be doing at least 9.3 miles a week. The training guidelines show you how to accomplish this. Be cautious in your training mileage. Run the race distance at least once in practice before you toe the starting line, even if it is just a fun run.

Here's how to do a 5K (3.1-mile) fun run or race:

1. Go back to your training chart by time.

2. If you can run:

- thirty minutes at a ten-minute-mile pace, you can run three miles right now. You can easily finish this race.

- thirty minutes at a twelve-minute-mile pace, you can run 2.5 miles right now. The thrill of the race will undoubtedly carry you through, but for your own confidence, you will want to build up so that you can run thirty-seven minutes, which is about the time you will need to cover 3.1 miles.

3. Continue to calculate based on your per-mile time.

Here's how to do a 10K fun run or race:

- If you can run thirty minutes at an eight-minute-mile pace, you can run nearly four miles (3.8 to be exact). You are quite fit, so building up to a 10K run will not be too difficult. See "Becoming a One-Hour Runner" on page 32; by week 8 you will have done sufficient training to complete the race. However, if you carry on with this program for the full ten weeks, the chances are that the increased mileage will make you stronger and faster by race time.

- If you can do thirty minutes at a ten-minute-mile pace, you can run three miles. You will need to be able to run for about sixty minutes at this pace to get through the event comfortably. See "Becoming a One-Hour Runner," page 32.

- If you can do thirty minutes at a twelve-minute-mile pace, you can run 2.5 miles. You will need to be able to run for about seventy-two minutes (this is one hour and twelve minutes) at this pace to get through the event. This is a long time to be on your legs, so you need to follow the instructions in "Becoming a One-Hour Runner," page 32, and add two more weeks to the program, increasing the time incrementally.

Note: all of these calculations are on the cautious side. Once you are in a fun run or race, the excitement and companionship of the event inevitably carry you through, even when you are shy of practice time and mileage. We all know of plenty of women who never ran more than three miles who easily completed a 10K run, or of a fitness walker who easily jogged a 5K race. But women over forty should take a conservative approach—make sure you do the proper training so as not to strain muscles, overheat a body that is not used to extra running time, or fatigue an untrained body.

TIP

As soon as you start calculating your mileage and times and start eyeballing a local running event, you'll be curious about how fast you can go or how much you think you can improve. See "Getting Faster," below. But remember, just doing it is what matters. Don't put pressure on yourself to become faster, and don't let anyone else push your pace unless you want him or her to. Husbands and boyfriends are notorious for doing this, not necessarily because they are trying to act superior (though sometimes they are), but because men in general run a lot faster than women. (To know why, see "Women and Men Running Together: Our Differences, Our Relationships," page 43.)

A personal note:

The thrill of a race or fun run brings out the best in you. Even when I am there just to jog along for fun and not racing at all, I am astonished at how much better I run in these situations. It also feels much easier—to do the times I do in a fun run would take a lot of effort in practice, and when I look back at my quality race times, I remember that I could never duplicate those in a training session. That's why I always like women to enter running events. It is fun and inspiring, and you always amaze yourself. Never discount the benefits of getting excited!

Getting Faster

The only way to get faster is to go faster! You cannot expect to run a four-mile fun run in twenty-four minutes (eight-minutes-per-mile pace) if you do all your training at ten minutes a mile. When it comes to speed, wishing won't make it happen. And no matter how old you are, you can remember a time when you ran too fast up the stairs or had to run hard in gym class and found yourself breathless and weak-kneed. It's not a comfortable feeling.

To run faster, you have to develop your heart to pump more blood, you have to train your lungs to transport more oxygen, and you have to condition your muscles to move faster and better utilize the blood and oxygen you're sending them.

Most of us want to go faster because faster is usually equated with being better. That is not always the case, and women in particular are discovering that the health benefits of running seven minutes a mile do not appreciably outweigh the benefits of running eight minutes a mile. In fact, for the beginning runner, quite the opposite is true. Fortunately, we usually know when we are going too fast—Mother Nature leaves us breathless.

A personal note:

For the average person, it is far better to run for a sustained period of time at a target heart rate than to try to go faster. That is why in this book I emphasize distance and routine over speed.

All things being equal, your target heart rate for exercise is when your heart is working at 60 to 80 percent of your maximum heart rate. (For details on determining your target heart rate, see page 22.) The general rule of fitness exercise is to keep moving for thirty minutes three times a week within this zone. Interestingly, the more you do it, the easier it is for your body to work efficiently. Soon you are able to go farther without raising your heart rate and without getting tired. You are also able to go faster because your heart, lungs, and muscles are all better trained and working more effectively. Only when you reach this stage should you attempt to go faster.

Interval Training/Speed Development Workouts

One of the easiest ways to get faster is to do speed work called intervals. You run faster for an interval of time and then rest for an interval of time. There are many different interval workouts favored by runners and coaches. Here are three that are fun and simple. Don't forget to do your normal warming up and cooling for the workout. Spend only one day a week on speed work. Speed training should be incorporated as a part of your normal workout time. If you run for forty minutes, just take a portion of that time for speed work.

1. Stride out faster than your normal pace, but don't sprint, for one minute. Then jog easily for one minute. Then stride out again for another minute. Start with three sets per session and work up to ten. Make sure you run for your full allotment of time during this session.

2. Stride for seventy-five seconds, rest/jog for forty-five seconds. Start with two sets and work up to ten sets.

3. Stride for one minute, rest/jog for one minute. Stride for two minutes, rest/jog for two minutes. Stride for two minutes, rest/jog for one minute. Stride for one minute, rest/jog for one minute. Begin with two sets and work up to four sets.

Getting Competitive:
The World of Masters Running

There is a whole new world out there for the over-forty woman who wants to be competitive as a runner. It's fun and it's exciting. It is also the only place in our society where men and women boast about their age, and where another birthday does not depress them but instead sends them out in pursuit of new races. This is the world of masters competition, as it is known in the United States, or veterans competition as it is known in the rest of the world.

These people compete within their age group and are awarded prizes based on performances against each other (and sometimes against international standards). Accurate records are kept and athletes vie to exceed them. Although the competition is friendly, it is also fierce. These masters runners and walkers consider themselves very serious athletes, and their performances are truly remarkable; many would stand up well in most of the road races in the United States.

It is a beautiful sight to see men and women, some well into their seventies and eighties, looking fit and healthy and enjoying movement as if they were teenagers and competing as ferociously as if they were Olympians. Many of them are indeed past Olympians who have a life-long affinity with fitness. Many more are people who never had the time or opportunity to be athletes before. And an ever-increasing number are people who discovered running or walking later in life and got hooked. Maybe you are one of them?

This group has more than proved the adage, "Use it or lose it." They are also the group that has proved more than any other that exercise is the secret to optimum weight and health. I've often said that if you put bags over their heads, you couldn't tell them from eighteen-year-olds!

The masters athletes are just beginning to get the respect they deserve, and that is not only because of an ever-increasing older population that has the disposable income to pursue fitness but also because these people are the cutting edge of what real fitness is: the lifelong commitment to a regular exercise program. They know there is nothing in life more important than health and happiness. Along the way, they've become, or stayed, very good at what they do. They can be an inspiration to you.

Regardless of your level of proficiency, you are welcome in almost any masters group. Like people in all kinds of fun runs and road races, they come from a huge variety of backgrounds and are open, welcoming, social, and proactive regardless of who you are. They are not cliquish. Despite many career accomplishments, most of them have made fitness the centerpiece of their lives and that is the common denominator.

A personal note:

Many a woman over forty experiences tremendous personal loss in her midlife years. The kids grow up and leave; she may feel that her looks and figure start to fade; her job plateaus; her romantic life is blah. Fight back! Running and walking are not only methods for reclaiming personal self-esteem; the whole masters running/walking movement is a tremendous source of rediscovery: new friends, new challenges, new places, and even new relationships.

Almost all running races on the road have a masters division for women. The age categories can be pretty competitive, but the friendships are great. Meeting men and women on your own might be difficult if you just show up alone at a race, so here are some suggestions:

- Join a local running or walking club and get to know the masters.
- Organize a masters-only running or walking clinic in advance of the local race.
- Go with an experienced masters runner or walker to an event and ask him or her to introduce you to others.
- Subscribe to *National Masters News*, the newspaper that covers

all aspects of masters running and walking from clubs to competitions. (See page 195 for the address.)

Here's a rundown of some of the best masters events.

WORLD MASTERS GAMES. More than thirty thousand participants from around the world compete in twenty-five sports, including a full schedule of running and walking events on the track and a marathon and a half marathon on the road. No time restrictions, and with so many athletes, there's no way you'll feel like the oldest, slowest, or fattest. An Olympic-style competition held every four years.

WORLD ASSOCIATION OF VETERANS (WAVA) CHAMPIONSHIPS. Held every two years, this is the world championships of over-forty running. Age categories are broken into five-year age groups. The winners are phenomenally good, but everyone is welcome. The cross-country (10K) and marathon are mass starts, so you won't feel as conspicuous as you would on the track with fast runners.

NATIONAL MUTUAL MASTERS GAMES, NEW ZEALAND. Held every other year alternating between Dunedin and Wanganui, New Zealand, this might be an excuse for the trip of a lifetime for you! Eight thousand athletes participate in sixty-seven different sports including a full program of running on the track and road for all abilities and in all over-forty age categories.

INDY LIFE MASTERS CIRCUIT. The Indianapolis Life Insurance Co. and USA Track and Field Association award points in nine races to several over-forty age groups. Includes races from distances of 5K to the marathon and awards $130,000 in prize money.

AVON RUNNING-GLOBAL WOMEN'S CIRCUIT. This series of eleven women-only 10K (and 5K fitness walks) races in the United States gives age group prizes for every five-year category from over forty through over eighty. Several of the sixteen international events also reward age groups. At its Global Championship prize money is awarded to at least the first three over-forty competitors.

If you'd like to know how you stack up against other women runners your age or convert your current running times compared to what you could have done in your prime years, say age twenty to thirty-four, it's now possible using tables you can order from *National Masters News.*

Women and Men Running Together: Our Differences, Our Relationships

Women and Men. We're so alike, and we're so different. Men are better at sports and fitness, right? No. Men are better at *some* activities, women at others. What's the difference? Men have more lean muscle mass and larger heart and lung capacity. This means that they can generally run faster, leap higher, and hit harder. They are also usually bigger than women, and bigger people are usually stronger than smaller people regardless of sex.

Men have also grown up with the sports, fitness, and regular athletic competition as part of their maturation process. It's not new to them, and they are most often not afraid of it.

Women are smaller, more flexible, carry more body fat, and have greater capacity for endurance. This doesn't mean they are not as good at sports or fitness; it means they are better in different ways. They can run longer, float more easily, endure cold better, and are better at stretching and flexibility exercises.

Women, who until recently have looked on from the sidelines of fitness activity, are often more receptive to new information, as well as willing to try new activities and training methods. Professional coaches say they love working with women because they are more coachable, without preconceived notions about how and what to do. Women are cautious at first, but it serves them well because by working gradually they avoid injuries. Weekend warrior injuries are almost all male!

If you want your partner along for help and tips, by all means run together, as long as you don't get competitive or contentious with each other. If he is constantly trying to outpace you, corrects your form, or generally makes you feel uncomfortable and tense, it's probably best for you just to go it alone. You'll both be happier in the long run.

If you run at the same pace and he is willing to let you shape your own program, training together can be extremely rewarding. When you run together, you have a tendency to talk things out and share thoughts, just like the inner conversations you have when you run alone. Sometimes you articulate thoughts you never could in a face-to-face, static situation. This new honesty and openness often is extremely therapeutic. If the relationship is new, it's a quick way to get to know a lot about each other. If running is a quiet time for you, that too can be shared.

A personal note:

> My husband runs much faster than I do but warms up as slowly as I do. We often start together and then separate. When we are in strange or remote places, we have an agreed-upon meeting place and time, and we never violate it. If I am anxious about an isolated running place or a difficult terrain, I'll ask my husband to turn back every twenty minutes on his run to check on me running behind him. It's all still running time, so it doesn't make a difference in the workout, and it frees me from worry. Actually, it frees us both, as it's a good check on each other in case of injury, too.

Running with a man affords many women a feeling of safety and can relieve a lot of the anxiety that results from running alone. This is particularly true for a beginner or anyone who regularly has to run in the dark.

Running together is extremely good in another very exciting way: When you exercise, your body secretes endorphins, which are natural mood enhancers. That's why during and after exercise you feel so good. When you exercise together, you feel good and come to associate those feelings with your partner. Plenty of marriages and relationships could benefit from this natural stimulant!

A personal note:

Running is wonderful, because you can do it anywhere. Whether you live in a city, the suburbs, or the country, there are roads, sidewalks, parks, and nature trails.

When you run for time, you just go out the door for half the time of your workout and then head back, retracing your steps. Sometimes total randomness is fun, and it's a great way to discover new sights. However, soon you will have your favorite routes.

In suburban Virginia, I have out and back courses that take from twenty minutes to two hours, along with various loops for variety and the odd five minutes I can tack onto a workout. I run on suburban roads, on sidewalks, in housing developments, on school fields, and on the marvelous Washington & Old Dominion bike trail—old railroad tracks that have been pulled up and replaced with a smooth asphalt bike/running/walking trail. I like it a lot because it's pretty and traffic-free.

In New York City, I run in Central Park. Morning or evening there are thousands of runners, roller bladers, and bikers in the park. Despite the bad news you hear about it, I am certain you are safer there than you are on a deserted road in the Midwest. It is a fabulous place to run or walk with loops of different lengths, plenty of hills, and lots of people-watching to make the time fly by.

While I was growing up in Virginia, going to college in upstate New York, and living in the Connecticut countryside, I did all my running on the sides of the road. Out in the country, there are not a huge number of cars, and I found the endless expanse of road exhilarating. But I also found it tiresome literally to have to leap off the road when I suspected a driver of being too close or too reckless.

Many of my runs were in the dark, and although I always wore reflective gear and moved well off the road when a car was approaching, many times I'd have to step into a ditch, a slushy snowbank, or a deep, muddy field to avoid being hit. If you have to run on roads, give traffic a wide berth.

Whenever I travel, I head out for a run at the first available opportunity to get a sense of where I am. Nothing comes close to running for making me feel quickly familiar with a strange place. I have seen some of the most incredible sights—Paris at night, Florence early in the morning, and dusty farm roads in central Illinois just before a thunderstorm—that tourists and couch potatoes never see.

Nowadays, there is a whole generation of women that is doing its running on treadmills. I have happily used a treadmill when it was too icy outside to run or late at night in a hotel in an unfamiliar city. While their usefulness is much greater than this, all things being equal I would always choose to combine my run with discovering the joys of nature, watching the world go by, and getting some fresh air.

chapter 4

A WALKING PROGRAM

A STEP-BY-STEP APPROACH TO A NEW WAY OF LIVING AND LOOKING GREAT

Walking is one of the most natural things we do. It's such a basic part of life that for a long time no one thought about it as a fitness activity. That's not the case anymore. As more and more people see the importance of exercise but are short on time, training, or even the ability to participate in more vigorous sports, they've decided to look elsewhere for a workout.

Fitness walking—walking with a purposeful stride, arms pumping, heart rate elevated—which first gained a following in the 1970s, is booming again as a result. It provides women with a wonderful exercise alternative. You can burn fat, develop muscle tone, reduce bone mass loss, and improve your grace and carriage.

Walking is going on everywhere: on the streets where you live, in community fun walks and races, through walking club activities, and

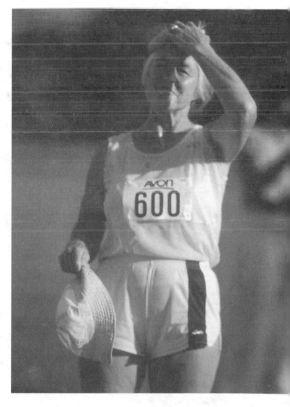

at shopping malls. You can walk anywhere, at almost any time. Most importantly, virtually everyone can walk, no matter what your current level of fitness or activity is.

If significant weight loss is a major goal for your exercise program, walking may be an excellent way to start. You use about 100 calories for every mile walked, more if you go faster. Best of all, walking raises the metabolism and thus keeps calories burning faster, even for awhile after you stop exercing.

Dr. Ayne Furman, a runner and podiatrist from Alexandria, Virginia, says that even if overweight women want to run, they should choose walking first. "Women with large thighs usually are forced to walk with their feet wide apart and thus they don't have a normal walking gait. It will be accentuated if they run, possibly leading to discomfort. So they are better off walking. If you lose twenty pounds, that generally translates to two inches off your thighs. At that point, you can try running." That is, if you are not already hooked on walking!

Just as there are progressive levels in running, there are different stages in walking. You may start by walking fifteen minutes, then work up to forty-five minutes three or four times a week to increase your fitness and develop a more healthful lifestyle. After feeling comfortable at that level, you may want to be more competitive and eventually train for and take part in races. Perhaps you've seen racewalkers during the Olympics or other large track meets and dream about doing that yourself someday in masters races, which feature competition in age groups starting at forty years old.

No matter what level you ultimately decide to reach for, everyone starts at the same place. We all know how to walk. How do you become a fitness walker? You do it by fitting your natural abilities into the framework of a walking program.

WALKING FORM Walk holding your body in a natural upright posture with your back straight, shoulders down, and neck relaxed. Look straight ahead, focusing three or four yards in front of you, not down on your feet.

Your heel should hit the ground first, then follow through your stride, pushing off with your toes. Hold your arms with your elbows bent at a 90-degree angle and pump them back and forth in an opposite rhythm to your feet—when you stride forward with your left foot, your right arm comes forward and vice versa.

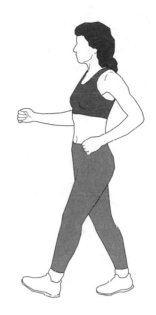

Keep your stride at a natural length. If you want to walk faster, don't lengthen your stride. Take smaller, quicker steps instead. Also, don't lean forward as you walk. Good posture not only enhances your carriage but also helps prevent injury.

A Program to Make You a Thirty-Minute Walker

Once you're able to walk comfortably for fifteen minutes, it's time to look at the next stage: working toward being a thirty-minute walker. This means you will be able to do a thirty-minute fitness walk three or four times a week. It's the stage at which many of your overall fitness goals will begin to be realized.

Start each walking session with a gentle warm-up walk for three or four minutes to loosen your muscles. After you finish your workout, cool down with a few more minutes of slow walking and then some gentle stretches (see page 19). The cooldown will relax your muscles and provide a smooth transition from your aerobic workout to your regular activities.

This program allows you gradually to build up to a thirty-minute walk over eight weeks. Not everyone will be able to do the program in that time. Follow the schedule at a comfortable pace but one that challenges you to move forward.

The program is based on the "hard-easy" training method. You make progress in training by pushing yourself to do more, but your body needs time to recover from the extra effort. The day after a hard workout when you walked faster or did extra mileage, schedule a day off, do an easier workout—less pace or mileage—or switch to an alternative type of exercise like biking, swimming, or strength training. Make it your goal to walk three or four times a week, but don't walk more than six days a week—give yourself a day off.

No one is judging you or holding you to a timetable. When you reach the point at which you can do a thirty-minute fitness walk as part of your regular routine, you'll have something that you can count on for the rest of your life. If it takes a little more time to get there, don't worry about it—you're in this for the long haul.

A personal note:

I can't stress enough the need for you to make a commitment to a routine, even though I also say not to feel guilty about missing a workout. If you know that you usually walk on Tuesday, Saturday, and Sunday, you focus on those days. When you think you can put it off for a day, you tend to start a pattern of procrastination. You miss days, mess up your schedule, and get discouraged. If it's on the calendar, you'll do it. And you'll be surprised that even when you think you're really tired, doing your walk energizes you!

WEEK 1: Walk 10 minutes, rest 3 minutes, walk 5 minutes. Rest 1 minute, then repeat.

WEEK 2: Walk 10 minutes, rest 1 minute, walk 5 minutes. Rest 1 minute again, then repeat.

WEEK 3: Walk 10 minutes, rest 1 minute, walk 10 minutes. Rest 1 minute, then repeat.

WEEKS 4 AND 5: Walk 20 minutes each session.

WEEKS 6 AND 7: Walk 25 minutes each session.

WEEK 8: Walk 30 minutes each session.

If you're comfortable after the first couple of weeks, you may want to speed up this timetable and complete the program in five or six weeks.

TIP

You should always be able to carry on a conversation while you're walking. If you can't, you're going too fast and should slow down.

Walking Farther and Faster: The Next Steps in Fitness Walking

After you've become a thirty-minute walker, you may simply want to continue to reap the benefits that accrue from that level of regular exercise. But if you want to go on to new goals and levels of accomplishment, there are attractive options open to you. Two of the most interesting are going faster and going farther. Increasing your speed and mileage gives you a more potent aerobic workout with its conditioning and fat-burning benefits. It can also keep your program fresh so your workouts don't become boring or routine.

Try to become a forty-five-minute or a one-hour walker by adding a longer walk to your regular program. Select one day on your workout schedule for a longer walk and gradually add ten-minute increments to your workout until you reach a comfortable and invigorating longer distance. Always schedule a day off after your long walk for rest and recovery.

Here's a four-week program to follow to become a sixty-minute walker. Bear in mind that these are only guidelines. It may take longer to reach the next level comfortably. Don't go ahead until you are ready.

WEEK 1: Walk three days for 30 minutes each session. Walk 40 minutes for the fourth session of the week.

WEEK 2: Repeat week-one schedule.

WEEK 3: Walk three days for 30 minutes each session. Walk 50 minutes for the fourth session.

WEEK 4: Repeat schedule for week 3.

WEEK 5: Walk three days for 30 minutes each session. Walk 55 minutes for the fourth session..

WEEK 6: Walk three days for 30 minutes each session. Walk 60 minutes for the fourth session.

A personal note:

Not only does walking feel good, but when you accomplish a distance, you are instinctively challenged to try to go farther. Many of us have never attempted this kind of physical test before. Once you know you can do it, you become curious about how much more you can do—and thrilled by the excitement of trying.

Once you've gone longer distances, your goal may be to go faster. I've been talking about time and not mileage in this walking program because it is a good starting point, and time is such a big issue in all our lives. To see how fast you are walking, determine your mile walking time on a measured path or a local high school track. Tracks may be the easiest to use since they are a standard 400 meters (440 yards) and four laps equal one mile. Do your regular warm-up, then time yourself for the mile. With that baseline, you can start to keep track of your time during workouts and chart your time in your walking diary. As you walk faster, you naturally also increase your distance as well as the aerobic effects of your workout. Once again, the key is do this gradually. No one is keeping a stopwatch on your workouts. Don't do too much too soon.

Getting Competitive: Finding the Fun in Racing

Once you can maintain your target heart rate by walking quickly for thirty minutes, not counting warm-up and cooldown, you are a serious walker. You can prove this to yourself by entering a 5-kilometer race—usually called a 5K—which covers 3.1 miles.

Racing is fun. You may get a T-shirt, meet other walkers, and gain the satisfaction of crossing the finish line just like all those athletes you've watched on television or in local races.

Start getting ready for your 5K by seeing how long it takes you to walk the 3.1 miles. Either use a track, a measured course, or one of your regular routes whose distance you are sure of and walk at your normal pace. If you do a sixteen-minute mile, it should take you just over forty-eight minutes to complete the 5K distance. If you walk at twenty-minute pace, it would take just over an hour.

Now that you know the time it takes you actually to cover the race distance, you can set up a training schedule, using the principles in this chapter, so you'll be ready for the event. If you don't normally walk three miles during your workouts, you can make building up to this distance your goal for the race and increase your distance through your workouts. If you do three miles regularly on your long walk, then you may want to work on your speed. In either case, give yourself sufficient time to reach your goal. And if you don't quite reach your goal, don't worry. There is always another race to participate coming up soon.

During the final week before the race, taper off your training for the last couple of days so you'll be well rested and eager to go on race day. Remember to have fun, raise your hands in triumph when you cross the finish line, and wear your new T-shirt the next day.

Walking in Indoor Spaces

Although walking indoors is not ideal, malls have emerged as an excellent place to walk for many reasons: convenience, time management, and safety. Malls provide a safe, weatherproof environment with plenty of amenities such as restrooms, benches, and water fountains. Walking in a mall represents an excellent use of time by allowing you to combine activities. If you're going to the mall to shop, see a movie, or have dinner, why not go a half hour or so earlier and do your fitness walk?

Many malls sponsor walking programs or clubs to encourage you to use their space. At the Mall of America in Bloomington, Minnesota, more than twenty-seven hundred women and men are members of Mall Stars, the center's walking club. Members receive a card that enables them to electronically track their mileage through the approximately 2.5 miles of floor space that make up the largest mall in the United States. In addition, there are training classes, shopping discounts, and programs on health and nutrition. The mall opens at 7:00 A.M. for walkers, but with its restaurants and movie theaters, the mall can accommodate walkers throughout the day and evening as well.

A similar program exists at Tysons Corner Center in McLean, Virginia, where mall walkers can use the facility before regular business hours. The club provides breakfast on the weekends, shopping discounts—and a lot of encouragement. Many malls around the country have similar programs. Contact the management office to get more information. If none of the malls near you offers a walking program, why not suggest that they start one?

Indoor walking has spread beyond the mall. Minneapolis and St. Paul are unique for their network of enclosed walkways between downtown buildings that helps people move about in their very cold winter. Now, in both cities, a coalition of businesses, civic groups, and health providers is sponsoring walking clubs to get workers out of the office and on the walkways for exercise during the day.

Racewalking: A Commitment to Athletics

Racewalking is an Olympic long-distance sport. Men have had Olympic racewalking competitions for decades at twenty kilometers

(12.4 miles) and fifty kilometers (31 miles). The Olympics opened racewalking for women in 1992 with a 10K event, and they now compete at 20K as well.

Although speed is the goal, and endurance, strength, flexibility, and overall conditioning are essential, technique is the essence of racewalking. The most elemental description of racewalking differentiates the event from running by the stipulation that there is unbroken contact with the ground—that is, one foot must always be on the ground; the forward foot must make contact before the rear foot leaves the ground. Furthermore, the leg in contact with the ground must be completely straightened on contact and remain straight until the body passes over the leg. Other components of racewalking form include bending the elbows at 85- to 90-degree angles and reaching forward with each hip to lengthen the stride.

Coaching is required to develop proper racewalking technique. You can get a good introduction to racewalking through videos or books (see the book list on pages 193 to 194). In New York, Howard "Jake" Jacobson, director of Walkers Club of America, pioneer promoter of racewalking and coach of Olympic racewalkers, conducts free weekly racewalking classes in Central Park and Long Island, year-round. On the West Coast, you can get excellent training from Elaine Ward, who operates the North American Racewalking Foundation from her home in Pasadena, California.

Walking Clubs and Masters Races: Places to Socialize and Compete

Among the offshoots of the growth in fitness walking is the development of walking clubs and, for those who want to test themselves competitively, masters races.

You don't have to wait until you're an accomplished fitness walker to join a club. In fact, the fellowship and information a club offers can be real boosts to your fitness efforts. Clubs may offer group walks and formal walking workouts. Members often share walking books and magazines as well as training information.

If there isn't a walking club in your area, join a running club. Most walkers are self-coached, anyway. A running club offers all the social benefits of a walking club. You have the companionship of like-minded people interested in health and fitness. There are also parties and club races in which you can participate or volunteer. Running clubs have full racing calendars. There is increasing respect for the run or walk option in races, and most accept people in three categories: runner, walker, and those who do a bit of both to get through the race.

Masters races offer a new world for over-forty walkers who want to test themselves in competition. With the possible exception of senior citizen discounts, it's one of the few places in our society where you're rewarded for getting older. Athletes compete against others in their age category with new competitive divisions for each decade starting at age forty.

Regardless of your level of expertise, you're welcome in almost any masters group. (See page 42 for a complete rundown of the major masters competitions.)

chapter 5

EQUIPMENT AND CLOTHING

FROM SHOES TO BRAS TO WATER BOTTLES, EVERYTHING YOU NEED (AND DON'T NEED) TO GET ON THE ROAD

Running and walking are the ultimate low-equipment sports. Just put on an old and comfortable T-shirt and pair of shorts, slip into your socks and shoes, open the door, and you're out there *doing it.* Unlike sailing, for instance, for which you need a boat as well as considerable time and money, running and walking are part of your everyday lives anyway, so making them part of your fitness program requires a minimum of fuss and bother.

However, low equipment doesn't mean there is no equipment required. You'll need a few basics: proper shoes, socks, and

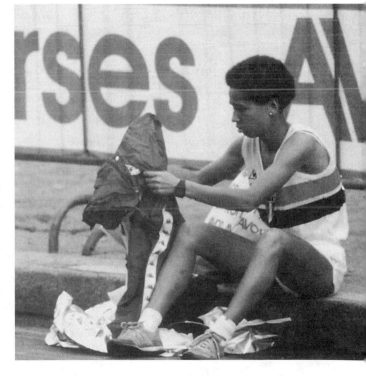

comfortable, nonrestrictive clothing and protection against the elements: sun, rain, and extremes in temperature. Today's fitness clothing industry recognizes the potential of the women's market and provides a tremendous number of clothing options. You can indulge a love of shopping and find fashionable and functional clothing for every taste and budget. Or you can mine your closets and drawers for comfy old things that you wouldn't wear anywhere else but are perfect for running and walking.

Clothing Essentials

All walkers and runners need a good pair of shoes and socks, loose clothing, and sunscreen for days and reflective gear for cloudy days or at night. In addition, a runner may need a sports or support bra. Whether to wear a bra and what type is best are two of the most vexing questions for women participating in all sports and for runners in particular. I'll discuss it in depth later in this chapter (page 77), but first let's look at the single most important piece of equipment you need, and the only one you'll have to go out and buy before getting started—shoes.

Buying the Right Shoe

Shoes are the *only* piece of *quality* equipment you need for walking and running. Why? The answer is in the numbers. When you walk or run a mile, your feet strike the pavement seventeen hundred times. During a thirty-minute walk or run that's a total of about four thousand times, and it increases to about six thousand times for a thirty-minute run. This pounding travels through the foot, up the ankle and knee, and into the hips and back. No wonder it's called "road shock."

Your shoes are your only protection against the constant striking of foot to ground. They absorb the shock and help keep your entire body in proper alignment, so you are less likely to wind up with problems in your knees, hips, or back. Getting the right shoe can make the fitness experience heavenly. Getting the wrong ones can make every step miserable and even cause injuries.

WHAT'S OUT THERE IN THE SHOE MARKET?

In 1980, you couldn't find a manufacturer making women's walking or running shoes! Although that might have been understandable in terms of walking—after all, walking was not yet widely recognized as a fitness exercise—it was incredible for running. The women's running boom began in the late 1970s, and there were thousands of registered women runners by 1980. So what did women do? They bought the smallest available sizes in men's running shoes—and suffered.

As we know too well, a woman's foot is different from a man's. Our foot is generally narrower, particularly in the heel. We are also more likely to have bunions, especially as we get older. These swollen, protruding joints at the base of the big toes are partly the price we're paying for too many years in tight, pointy-toe shoes and high heels, though more commonly they are the result of inheriting a predisposition to develop bunions.

Although women's feet pose challenges to proper fit, the good news is that shoe manufacturers have awakened to the large market for women's running shoes. So today's female runners no longer have to wear scaled-down versions of men's shoe. The shelves are stocked with shoes designed to fit a women's foot.

As walking took off as a fitness activity in the 1980s, women dominated the sport, and shoe manufacturers started producing a wide array of shoes designed specifically for us. It's now a multimillion-dollar market and one where women overshadow men as both participants and consumers.

Before going to the store or mall to buy shoes, here's a game plan to follow that will ensure you get the proper shoes and help you to shop with confidence.

GOLDEN RULES FOR SHOE BUYING

RULE 1. BE PREPARED TO SPEND $60 TO $90 FOR THE CORRECT PAIR OF SHOES. You may be lucky and find good ones on sale, but don't expect it. Trust me: The right shoes are worth every penny.

RULE 2. BUY ONLY TO FILL YOUR SPECIFIC NEED. Proper walking or running shoes are not designed for tennis or aerobics. Don't think one pair of shoes can be used for all sports. It can't.

RULE 3. DON'T BE INFLUENCED BY LABELS OR PRICE. A chic designer label, a heavily promoted manufacturer's name, and shoes with price tags that start at $125 and up are very misleading for a beginner, who might think that name and price guarantee quality. Read on.

A personal note:

Even after running for thirty-seven years, I have to brace myself when I go to buy new shoes because the selection is so overwhelming and the technology is changing every six months. Plus I hate to spend a lot of money I can't afford to waste on the wrong choice. Hey, I've never spent $90 on even a pair of everyday shoes in my life! I really don't want to make a mistake. That's why I always rely on experts who earn their living selling quality shoes and fitting them.

RULE 4. PROPER FIT IS ESSENTIAL. Buy your shoes from a specialty walking or running store, where the salespeople are trained to fit walkers and runners—they generally are walkers and runners themselves. They will ask questions about your program, your aspirations, your particular foot twinges and aches. Then they'll check your foot type and watch as you walk and run in the shoes you try on. They can steer you away from making choices based on name or image. The fitters in these stores are an invaluable resource for you. Use them. If you sense that the person helping you is a rookie, don't be embarrassed to do a little comparative shopping elsewhere, or to come back on a different day.

Avoid catalogs and huge sports megastores until you know what you're buying.

RULE 5. DON'T BE SCARED OFF BY TECHNICAL TERMS LIKE "PRONATION" OR "SUPINATION." They each mean something simple, and a good fitter will explain these terms and others. To further educate yourself before you hit the store, see "Tech Talk About Running Shoes," page 63.

RULE 6. DON'T TRY TO SELECT SHOES WHEN YOU'RE IN A HURRY. Buying the proper shoes takes time: You need to try different styles, move around in them, and talk to the fitters. In terms of comfort and pleasure, it's worth all the time you spend.

RULE 7. PROPER FIT IS ALWAYS MORE IMPORTANT THAN TECHNOLOGY. Shoe manufacturers try to impress you with the latest flashy bells and whistles on various shoe models. Ignore most of them. This is another time when a good salesperson can make a difference. He or she can explain to you the *minimal* differences between things like gel or air or tell you when something is simply a marketing gimmick.

RULE 8. BRING YOUR ORTHOTICS WITH YOU WHEN YOU GO TO BUY RUNNING OR WALKING SHOES. If you are already wearing orthotics in your regular shoes, you will need to wear them while you are running or walking. Talk with your podiatrist about your plans to starting running or walking, so he or she can make a recommendation about the type of orthotic you should wear during exercise. It might be the same one you are already wearing or perhaps a new one specifically designed for exercise.

RULE 9. FOLLOW THE RULE OF THUMB. Try a variety of the recommended shoes and, while standing, check to be sure there is at least one thumb's width of space between the end of your longest toe and the front end of the shoe. This might be the single most important factor, since the shoe size you need for walking or running is often one size or more larger than your usual shoe size.

A personal note:

For most of my competitive running career, I suffered painful black toenails. This comes from the end of the toes banging into the front of the shoe, forming blood blisters underneath the toenails. It was years later that I found out that running shoes should not fit snugly. So be sure to allow for a full thumb's width between your longest toe and the end of the shoe. And keep your toenails trimmed.

RULE 10. DON'T FORGET YOUR SOCKS. Your shoes and socks need to work as a team. Discuss your sock needs with your salesperson and try on both the new shoes and socks you'll be wearing. This is particularly important if you need thickly cushioned socks. (See the section on socks, page 69.)

RULE 11. TAKE THE SHOES FOR A WALK OR RUN OUTSIDE THE STORE. A specialized athletic shoe store lets you take shoes out for a test walk or run since they know you can't determine fit and comfort by a few seconds of walking or jogging around in the store. The shoes should feel good right away. If they are uncomfortable and you think they need breaking in, they don't fit properly—make another choice. If these are your first athletic shoes, they probably will feel bulky compared to your dress pumps or casual flats.

RULE 12. WHILE WALKING OR RUNNING IN THE NEW SHOES, HAVE SOMEONE WATCH YOUR FEET. Either a friend or your salesperson can see how you are landing on the soles of the shoes. No matter how your foot outline looked during the wet test (page 63), you need to see exactly how your foot is reacting to a particular shoe in a live demonstration to be sure you're choosing the right one.

TECH TALK ABOUT RUNNING SHOES

As you know, shoes are designed to protect you against the deleterious effects of road shock and help place your body in proper alignment while running and walking. But how can you find the shoe that will accomplish both these tasks?

First, you need to find out what type of foot you have. The easy to do this is to take the "wet test." Wet your foot, shake off excess water, and step with your full weight onto a paper towel. Step away from the towel and hold it up to the light. You've created an impression of your foot—just like the dentist does of your teeth—that enables you to judge which of the three basic foot categories you fall into: *normal, flat,* or *high-arched.*

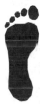

A normal foot (above) strikes the ground on the outside of heel and then rolls slightly inward to absorb shock. It's considered the most efficient stride and requires a *moderately controlling* shoe that provides stability for the foot.

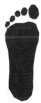

A flat foot strikes the ground on the outside of the heel and rolls inward excessively after landing. The excessive inward rolling is called pronating, and if you have this foot type, you need a *motion-control* shoe to keep you from continuing to pronate.

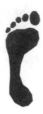

With a high-arched foot, when you hit the ground you stay on the outside of your foot instead of having the ideal slightly inward, shock absorbing roll. Sports podiatrists call this a supinated or underpronated foot. You will need a *cushioned shoe* that promotes the proper inward roll to produce an efficient and healthy stride.

TECH TALK ABOUT WALKING SHOES

If you were to watch a slow motion film of runners and walkers, it would quickly be apparent that the stride pattern for each is very different. Walkers step forward and always land on their heel, their weight rolls forward onto the ball of the foot, and then they push off. Depending on their speed, runners can land on their heel, midfoot, or, if they are running very fast, on the ball of their foot before pushing off. Since walkers spend more time and absorb most of their weight on their heels, walking shoes must have densely cushioned heels that absorb shock. Walking shoes also offer protection against excessive inward or outward foot rotation.

Although they share many of the same features, running shoes typically are thicker in the midsole, while walking shoes are cushioned evenly throughout the sole. Running shoes are not recommended for walkers, unless you are planning to use walking as a first stage in your running program.

With the variety of walking shoes available, it's just as important for a walker to be certain of her foot type before shopping. Take the "wet test" described above for runners to determine your foot type.

The following chart shows the three basic running and walking shoe categories and the types of runners who should use them. Bring it along when you buy your shoes. Discuss your foot type and each of these choices with the salesperson.

SHOES

Foot type	Stride	Best Running Shoe	Best Walking Shoe	Avoid	How Shoes Will Feel at First
NORMAL	Lands on outside of heel, rolls slightly inward. Considered most efficient foot; absorbs shock.	STABILITY shoe, such as Nike Air Pegasus, Reebok Interval, Saucony Grid Jazz and Grid Shadow, Asics Kayano	STABILITY shoe, such as Reebok Road Glider DMX, Rockport ProWalker World Tour, Nike Air Essential, New Balance 551	Cushioned or motion-control shoes that will decrease the efficiency of your running or walking stride.	A bit "boxy," then so comfortable you won't feel as if you are wearing anything.
FLAT	Lands on outside of foot then rolls inward excessively. Constant inward turning can result in overuse injuries.	MOTION-CONTROL shoe, such as New Balance 586, Nike Air Structure II, Asic Gel MC Plus, Brooks Addiction II, Etonic Stable Air Pro III, Brooks Beast	MOTION-CONTROL shoe, such as New Balance 840, Nike Air Provider RW, Wilson TW4040 CS, Rockport Motation, Etonic Pro Support	Cushioned shoes that will increase pronation problem and could cause injuries.	Takes a few wearings to get used to, then you'll feel inseparable.
HIGHLY ARCHED	Lands either on outside of heel, midfoot, or on balls of feet, but does not roll inward enough. This foot type is not an effective shock absorber.	CUSHIONED shoe with plenty of flexibility to encourage foot motion, such as Reebok Run DMX, Nike Air Max, Air Max Tailwind, or Air Max Triax, Adidas Equipment Light, Saucony Grid Hurricane, Fila Silva Trainer	CUSHIONED shoe, Such as Nike Air Sertive Max, Asics Gel-Savali II, Nike Air, Healthwalker LX, Adidas Solo II	Motion control shoes, which will restrict the flexibility and motion you need.	Wonderful. You'll wonder why you didn't always wear them.

PERFORMANCE SHOES: WHAT'S THE DIFFERENCE?

Once you become hooked on running and walking, simply keeping fit may not be enough. The lure of local, charity-sponsored runs and annual big races with their medals and T-shirts can turn even the most noncompetitive person into an intrepid racer. And once you've started to run or walk fast, why not try to go faster? If you do, you may eventually need a performance shoe in addition to your training shoe.

There are basically two kinds of performance shoes: lightweight trainers and racing shoes. No matter what their competitive level is, all runners and walkers spend most of their workout time training. While racking up mileage in preparation for a race, runners and walkers expect their shoes to protect them from injury, just as any beginner or fitness exerciser does. But racers also want a shoe with less weight so they can go faster. Lightweight trainers are the answer. They are lighter than regular training shoes but still can correct the tendency to pronate or supinate. They are also an ideal competition shoe for fast runners who need more support than racing shoes provide, or middle of the pack runners who want to improve their speed.

Racing shoes are a different story. Elite racers want to move quickly with a minimum amount of weight on their feet. The shoes of Olympic-level sprinters are as thin and delicate as ballet slippers—but with spikes on the bottom. Shoes worn by elite distance runners, who race several miles, have thin foam soles. Racing shoes provide almost no protection against road shock and are designed only for competition, while competitive racewalkers wear lightweight shoes with some cushioning and support.

TIP

SHOULD A WOMAN EVER BUY A MAN'S SHOE?

For years this was our only option. But today almost all men's training shoes are manufactured in equivalent women's models. However, few women's shoes come in a variety of widths, so if you require a wider shoe, as I do, consider trying on men's models as well as women's. The situation is different for racing shoes. Although they are labeled unisex, the sizes are actually based on men's shoe charts. Few companies make racing shoes exclusively for women, so for racing you may need to buy a man's shoe.

TAKING CARE OF YOUR SHOES

Your running and walking shoes are passports to a new lifestyle. They will take you to places you have never been before—and that will mean plenty of sweat, rain, mud, sand, and some doggy-do as well. Although you won't like getting the most expensive shoes you own dirty and smelly, it's inevitable. Some routine maintenance will keep your shoes relatively clean and odor-free.

After *every* run or walk, air out your shoes. The dampness caused by your feet sweating inside your shoes causes odor. The only way to get rid of it is to let your shoes dry out completely. If you wear heel pads, arch supports, or orthotics, take them out after exercising and let them dry separately. The manufacturer's insole should also be removed, so it can dry out as well. Put a sheet of scented fabric softener in each shoe to help them smell fresher.

When your shoes get soaked by rain or wet from running or walking through water, stuff them with old newspaper and let them dry away from heat. After a couple of hours, change the newspaper. When the shoes feel damp, remove the paper and open up the shoes as much as possible to let air get inside to finish the drying process. If the shoes are coated with mud, remove the mud with a stiff brush after the shoes are dry.

For some women, well-worn, grubby-looking sports shoes are evidence of good workouts. But if you want your shoes to look really clean, hose them off, then scrub them with a soapy brush, and quickly rinse off the soap. *Don't put your shoes in the washer and dryer.* They'll be clean, but the combination of water, soap, and heat will break down the integrity of the shoe's materials and you'll soon be needing a new pair of shoes.

A personal note:

My dirty running shoes fill me with joy. They've taken me over farm fences in Illinois, through streams in Colorado, rain forests in New Zealand, and on manure-covered bridle paths in England. They are my passports to freedom and my license to revisit my childhood. When I look at my running shoes, I see the steps of my past and the pathway to my future.

HOW OFTEN DO YOU NEED NEW SHOES?

Generally, runners and walkers change shoes every 400 to 500 miles, or every year if you run or walk three times a week. Although external wear is not the only indication you need new shoes, it's a good place to start. Some obvious signs of wear are worn treads on the sole, breaking down of the heel, or sliding over the sole during your run or walk. Walkers generally have greater wear in the front of the sole because of their stride. Also, depending on how you land, the heel may wear down sooner than the mileage guideline. If you see signs of wear, don't wait—replace your shoes.

Inspecting the inside of the shoe is crucial, as well. Shoes can deteriorate on the inside and need replacement even if the outside still looks wearable. If foam materials start to go flat, you can lose bounce and shock absorption. A good sign of a "dead" shoe is if the road or sidewalk suddenly feels very hard.

TIP

To be sure you don't wear the same old pair of shoes too long, use permanent ink to write the date you buy them on the heel. Then you'll know when to replace them.

Socks: The Second Most Important Piece of Equipment You Need

Shoes and socks—a natural combination, but one that's often taken for granted. We buy shoes carefully, then add socks as an afterthought, which can be a costly mistake in terms of comfort and pleasure. Socks protect your feet against the friction and sweat produced during exercise. To do the job, they should have smooth seams and fit correctly without wrinkling, sliding down your heel, or binding your toes.

Your favorite old pair of 100 percent cotton athletic socks are *not* up to the task. Cotton socks will absorb the moisture you produce during a run or walk, but they will also become ropelike and uncomfortable, providing the perfect environment for developing blisters. Today, socks made of synthetic fibers, or combinations of cotton, wool, and synthetics, reduce this risk by drawing moisture away from your feet and keeping it away, so you feel comfortable and dry throughout your run or walk. Socks also come in a variety of thicknesses with extra cushioning at pressure points such as the heel and toes. However, thicker socks take more space, so you may need a larger shoe size if you require extra protection in those areas.

A personal note:

It took me years of blisters, pain, and experimentation to get the correct socks. Finally, technology saved me with fabulous, nearly blister-free synthetics. While I cannot run without my thin CoolMax socks, my husband can train for miles and miles in nylon dress socks, and many walkers find thick wool socks ideal. Do what feels best for you. Keep trying different socks until you find the thinnest sock that feels snug but not tight around your feet.

Clothing

With the exception of shoes and socks, chances are you already have somewhere in your closets or drawers everything you need to start running or walking. As you get more proficient and begin looking for clothes for special conditions (rain, cold, extreme heat), you may want to purchase new things.

For both walkers and runners, the emphasis must be on comfort, mobility, and breathability. Don't wear anything that is the slightest bit restrictive. Scratchy materials, raised seams, and tight-fitting shorts or tops will irritate your skin once you start moving. Whether you are a beginner or an elite runner, chafing is a killer, and you'll find yourself turning to reliably comfortable garments time and time again when you're getting ready to start a workout. (See antichafing products on page 88.)

The clothes you wear for running or walking on any given day are largely determined by the weather. Is it hot or cold, windy or calm, sunny or cloudy, misty or raining, or somewhere in between? There are good choices for each.

A personal note:

Nothing is quite so joyful as making the first tracks in snow or being a part of the changing seasons. And nothing makes you feel quite as smug and superior as a workout in adverse conditions. With the right combination of clothing, you can always stay comfortable, so weather should almost never deter you from running or walking.

CLOTHING BASICS

Warm or Mild Temperatures

A beginning walker should wear loose, well-worn cotton shorts long enough to prevent thighs from rubbing and with plenty of room in the legs and crotch; a comfortable 100 percent cotton T-shirt with plenty of room around and under the arms; and your most comfortable and absorbent underwear. The ideal outfit for the beginning runner is the same as for a walker, except you should wear running shorts, tights, or bicycle-style shorts for greater comfort during your workout.

Cool Days

Walkers should replace shorts with loose running pants or tights (runners may wish to, as well, although shorts may still be enough), and a long-sleeve T-shirt or turtleneck. A lightweight warm-up suit is a good alternative for walkers, but it's too warm for runners, who still generate a lot of heat even on cool days.

Cold, Rainy Days

Add a water-resistant rain and wind top, preferably one that hangs over your hips, to your cool-weather outfit. A baseball cap is useful for keeping rain off your face and your head warm. Gloves are also needed.

You have to balance comfort and cost when you select a rain outfit. The choice is wide: from an inexpensive nylon windbreaker and pants to more expensive blends of polyester, nylon, or Gore-Tex. Nylon by itself is not a breathable fabric, so it can make you feel very hot and sweaty during your run or walk. The more expensive synthetic blend fabrics, which are lightweight, breathable, and waterproof, may justify their higher prices because they can be used even when you are not running or walking. (Consult the clothing chart on page 73 for styles and fabrics.)

Very Cold Days

Runners and walkers need a warm-up suit with tights, a turtleneck, and a thermal undershirt. It is essential to wear a hat and gloves. If you live in an extremely cold climate, you may want to consider purchasing a winter-weight Gore-Tex or similar running or walking suit. These are expensive but extremely durable and have many useful features such as built-in reflective strips. They are also excellent for casual wear.

A CLOSE-UP LOOK AT CLOTHING

As you get more proficient in your running and walking and more confident about your public appearance, you may want to get out of those loose shorts and into some of the sleek and attractive exercise wear you see in stores and on other runners and walkers. To help you navigate among the many choices in style and fabric, here are charts showing what's available in tops, pants, and warm-ups and their ideal uses.

SHORTS AND PANTS

Garment	Fabric Choices	Running Usefulness	Walking Usefulness	Features and Fashion	Advantages	Disadvantages
Running shorts	Nylon, CoolMax, Dri-F.I.T., supplex	Basic warm-weather bottom. Allows freedom of movement. CoolMax, supplex, or other synthetic fabrics are more comfortable than cotton or nylon.	Excellent choice in warm weather. Nonrestrictive for high-energy exercise.	CoolMax or other wicking fabrics used for built-in underpant. Select shorts with underpants that don't have elastic touching the skin. Long cut in the rear for more backside coverage.	Lightweight, total freedom of motion, built-in underpant; small pockets to hold keys and change.	All styles of shorts are very revealing. Larger, floppier shorts can bunch up in crotch.
Fitness shorts Bicycle shorts	Supplex, Lycra, cotton blend, combination fabrics	Fitness shorts made of combination fabrics give snug fit without chafing or seam marks. Total freedom of movement. Outstanding comfort.	Comfortable, snug-fitting shorts for energetic walk.	Bright fashion colors, very athletic look.	Highly flexible; soft fabrics; very lightweight and nonrestrictive, nonchafing.	Glove-tight fit, very revealing. True cycling shorts have thick protective pads—find running or walking versions of this look.
Midlength shorts (3–4" inseam)	Microsupplex	Good loose short.	Flexible, loose-fitting workout short.	Style is flattering to all figure types. Wide range of colors and prints. Doubles as a casual wear short.	Cotton is excellent for walking. Supplex blends are quick drying, useful for all-weather wear. Covers thighs fully. Drawstring waist offers better fit.	Runners may find these shorts too floppy for long runs. All-cotton versions are not good for runners.

Garment	Fabric Choices	Running Usefulness	Walking Usefulness	Features and Fashion	Advantages	Disadvantages
Tights Capri tights	Cotton, Lycra blend, supplex, polypropylene	Good cool-weather bottom.	Comfortable cool-weather bottom.	Very versatile exercise pant. Can be flattering for all figures with the right top. Capri tights are an older style finding a a new fashion spotlight.	Almost totally prevents chafing. Supplex blends feel soft and provide warmth for runners and walkers on cool or even cold days. High Lycra content offers lots of support, so you don't jiggle. Combines with long T to hide figure flaws.	Can be revealing if worn with a bra top or crop top. High Lycra content can feel somewhat restrictive.
Training pants	Polyester, nylon, Lycra blends	Short, easy runs.	All types of walking	Drawstring waist, deep pockets, leg zippers to make taking on and off over shoes easier. Soft, easy fit makes training pants an all-purpose sports, casual, and travel wear item.	Wind and dampness protection keeps you warm on slow runs and all walks. Good for warming up before a race and to keep from being chilled after a workout. Alternative to figure-revealing tights.	Inhibits rapid leg movement; not intended for fast workouts. Heats up quickly. May cause chafing on long runs or walks.

WARM-UPS, SWEATSUITS, AND RAIN AND COLD GEAR

Garment	Fabric Choices	Running Usefulness	Walking Usefulness	Features and Fashion	Advantages	Disadvantages
Sweatsuits/ Warm-ups	Nylon or poly/cotton blends	Cold-weather running, warming up before a race.	Cool and cold-weather walking.	Pockets with zippers, cotton or CoolMax liners, zip leg pants. Colorful, utilitarian sports outfit used as much for casual wear as exercise.	Loose and comfortable jacket and top. Can be tied around waist if you get too warm.	Usually too warm and bulky for running. Will chafe during long workouts.
Rain suits, breathable and non-breathable	Nylon or polyester, reinforced to be waterproof	Cold, soaking rains.	Cold, soaking rains.	CoolMax or cotton webbing lining. Covered zippers, including over pockets. Hood that laces tightly. Front zipper that closes up to chin. Bright colors and reflective strips or patches. Made with breathable fabric.	Breathable fabric used in combination with appropriate liners, will keep you dry during hard, cold rains. Dries quickly. Folds flat for easy packing on trips.	Those made of nonbreathable fabric builds up sweat and steam inside of suit; feels like you're working out in a greenhouse. Danger of overheating if worn in warm weather. Must be worn with a liner to prevent chafing. Fabric not flexible, need to wash carefully.
Cold weather and rain suit	Gore-Tex, Polartec, STORM-F.I.T. nylon. (You can also create your own cold-weather suit using a nylon rain suit worn with supplex or cotton pants, a turtleneck shirt, and an old old sweater or Polartec top.)	Extremely cold weather.	Extremely cold weather.	Zippers on pockets and legs. Long jacket to cover hips. Tab fasteners at cuffs and ankles to ensure tight fit. Hood that stores in roll collar and laces tightly. Draft protector at neck. Bright color and reflective strips or patches.	Very protective garment that allows you to work out in extreme cold. Add layers to stay outside for long runs or walks Washes and dries quickly. Long lasting. A Gore-Tex or other specialty fabric suit prevents moisture buildup during workout to keep you from getting wet and dangerously cold.	All outfits are expensive. Can make fast workouts less comfortable because suits are bulky. Very warm; shouldn't be worn in mild weather.

TOPS AND T'S

Garment	Fabric Choices	Running Usefulness	Walking Usefulness	Features and Fashion	Advantages	Disadvantages
Singlet Tank top Crop top	CoolMax, cotton, supplex, Dri-F.I.T., nylon, combination fabrics	Singlets are mainstay of running and racing wardrobe in hot weather; used by racers in almost any season. Tank and crop tops also great for warm weather.	Excellent hot weather tops; Singlet is the choice for racing.	Quick-drying fabrics. Singlets traditionally cut on a man's model with generous armholes and loose fit; combine with colorful bra top for a fashion look. Tanks tuck into shorts for loose fit. Crop tops cut above the waist allow plenty of air circulation.	All three tops made with CoolMax or combination fabrics keep you cooler in hot weather and warmer in cold weather; great travel choices, pack easily, wash and dry quickly.	In hot weather tops made from nylon dry stiff and can chafe. In high humidity, cotton gets soggy and heavy; also uncomfortable because wet stays on your body a long time.
Bra tops	Cotton/poly/ Lycra; CoolMax lining, supplex	Can be worn alone or under singlets.	Worn alone or under singlets.	Great colors; does double duty as bra and top; coordinates with shorts; very hip look.	Colorful breast support; cool when worn alone; CoolMax lining keeps moisture off skin.	Can feel tight and restrictive; some may cause chafing; very revealing when worn alone.
T-shirt Short sleeve Long sleeve	Cotton; polyester; 50/50 cotton and polyester blend; thick and thin weaves	CoolMax, thermax thermastat, or polypropylene fabrics are perfect for cool days—temperature under 65 degrees.	CoolMax, thermax thermastat, or polypropylene fabrics for excellent for moderate temperatures—under 75 degrees.	Traditional sports top; fun to wear to advertise your last race.	Oversize T's terrific cover-ups, particularly over figure-revealing shorts and tights; good post-workout top to replace sweaty garments.	When 100% cotton T gets wet, leaves moisture on your body, which can be uncomfortable.
Base layers: Thermalayer Turtle (In Sport); Dri-F.I.T. Piqué Basic shirt (Nike); Lightweight Drylete Crewneck (Hind); Lightweight Thermax Mode Turtle (Lioness)	Dri-F.I.T.; bipolar 100 or 200 polyester; polyolefin; polyester; polyester, Lycra, and nylon blends; polypropylene	Wear under jackets or vests, fits snugly to provide warmth and soak up moisture. Can be worn alone but works best as a bottom layer.	Wear under jackets or vests, fits snugly to provide warmth and soak up moisture.	Quick drying. Generally does not retain body odor. Many include zipper turtlenecks for adjustable air circulation. Lioness comes in a variety of beautiful colors; most are basic black, white, or gray. Variety of weights and thicknesses available for use in different weather conditions. Great under scratchy sweaters, too.	Essential for cold weather; wicking action allows body body to dry without feeling cold; Frictionless.	Need to select proper weight shirt depending on weather conditions to get best results.

GLOSSARY OF FABRICS

Over the past few years there's been a revolution in the manufacture of fabrics designed for active-wear clothing. Newly developed synthetic fibers keep you cooler in hot weather and warmer in cold weather by absorbing sweat as it develops on your body and drawing it away from your skin, so it has a chance to evaporate. This process is called "wicking." As a result of wicking, you don't have to suffer the heavy, clammy sensation of sweat-soaked cotton or the steamy feeling of nylon as you run or walk.

Many of these fabrics are made of polyester, a dreaded word to exercisers who associate it with the hot, unbreathable T-shirts they used to wear. Today, polyester has been transformed into a soft, breathable, wicking fabric that bears little resemblance to its former incarnation. But if you still have some T-shirts that are 50-50 cotton and polyester, leave them in your dresser when it comes time to run or walk.

The following glossary will familiarize you with the most common of these new fabrics and how they work.

COOLMAX: A 100 percent polyester fabric made of a four-channel fiber that provides 20 percent more surface area than average fibers to increase moisture transfer away from your skin to the outer layers of the fabric. There, the sweat evaporates so the fabric doesn't become waterlogged and your skin feels dry. CoolMax is also breathable, so you also get a steady flow of air through the fabric.

DRI-F.I.T., DRILAYER, AND DRYLETE: Three trademarked fabrics that use two-layer construction to transfer moisture from the layer against your skin to the top layer, where it can quickly evaporate. All provide excellent wicking properties.

FLEECE: A 100 percent polyester fabric known most widely as Polartec. It provides nearly the same warmth as wool but is quick drying, lightweight, durable, and washable. Polartec comes in several weights that can be used either as outer or middle layers.

GORE-TEX: A nylon fabric that provides excellent insulation without letting you overheat. This waterproof, breathable fabric allows water and vapor to escape but keeps wind and rain out.

LYCRA SPANDEX: A form-fitting, very stretchable material that is often combined with other fabrics to make them more comfortable and sleek looking.

POLYPROPYLENE: Provides outstanding insulation in cold weather when used as a first layer under a shirt and jacket. Polypropylene traps warm air against skin and wicks moisture away through upper layers of clothing.

SUPPLEX: A 100 percent nylon yarn made of more numerous and finer strands than ordinary nylon. As a result, supplex is lightweight, durable, breathable, and as soft as cotton on your skin. It is often combined with Lycra in shorts and tights.

Finding the Right Bra

Sports bras have definitely gone mainstream. Today, they combine fashion with function and are meant to be seen as well as support. On hot summer days, women sometimes discard singlets and T-shirts to run in sports bras alone—that's about as cool as you're likely to get in all senses of the word. Better-quality bra construction has also allowed larger-breasted women to run comfortably, perhaps for the first time.

However, buyer beware. Just because it looks like a sports bra and has a label that says it's a sports bra doesn't always mean you're buying something more functional than a colorful sun top. And while the technology of sports bras improves every year, they are far from perfect.

Nothing is more challenging to sports clothing designers than protecting the breasts against the hard, repetitive jarring and bouncing of running. Most running bras are designed on the simple principle that binding breasts keeps them from bouncing. If you want less bounce, make the binding tighter. But there is a price to be paid for this control. These bras require more fabric and heavier construction, and they definitely feel more restrictive than nonsports bras. The additional material also limits heat dissipation and some women may feel it limits their ability to breathe freely, although it actually doesn't.

There is no single answer to the question of what bra you should wear. Size and comfort are the keys. Whatever your size, you must find the bra that makes you feel most comfortable. Talking with other women who are your size and who have found a satisfactory bra is probably the best way to get reliable information about how a particular bra feels and wears. Shop around and try on many different bras. *Runner's World* magazine compiled the following bra chart that provides an excellent rundown of the most widely distributed bras and their features.

BRAS

Bra	Fabric	Sizes	Evaluation	Rating*
Action Tech, Champion	Outer layer: cotton and polyester; inner layer: CoolMax and Lycra spandex	Small–extra large	Fabric is soft and lightweight; provides excellent support. Elastic band around the chest prevents chafing.	Four stars in all categories.

Bra	Fabric	Sizes	Evaluation	Rating*
Dawn Sport, Dawn Lane	Nylon and Lycra for both inner and outer layers	Small—large	Best for runners and walkers who don't need a lot of support. Hand-sewn seams are very smooth and comfortable. Comes in array of prints and colors. Can be worn alone without a cover. Colors may bleed in washing.	Four stars for comfort; three stars for breathability and support.
Elitist, InSport	Supplex and Lycra blend; CoolMax and Lycra lining	Small extra large	Very comfortable; best for small to medium sizes. Variety of styles that provide equal comfort. Comes in many colors and prints.	Four stars for breathability and comfort; three stars for support
Endurance T-Top, IIind	Heavyweight nylon and Lycra with spandex	Small—large	T-back design and stretchy Lycra provide good support. Feels exceptionally soft next to skin.	Four stars for support; three stars for breathability and comfort.
Minimal Bounce, Sporteze	Mostly cotton, with Lycra to provide support	Small—extra large	Best for cotton lovers. Does not have strong moisture wicking properties. Shape, thin straps, and thin elastic band around bottom add to comfort. A bra you will either love or hate.	Four stars for comfort; three stars for support; two stars for breathability.
Olympia, Moving Comfort	Polyester, cotton, Lycra outer layer; lined with CoolMax and Lycra, nylon tricot stabilizers in straps for support	Small—extra large	Racer back construction offers excellent support, even for larger breasted women. CoolMax inset panel wicks moisture in front and arch-back opening increases ventilation.	Five stars for comfort; four stars for breathability and support.

Bra	Fabric	Sizes	Evaluation	Rating*
Sweat It Out, Lontex Corp.	CoolMax and Lycra	32A–40D (custom orders for larger sizes)	The lightest and most breathable bra tested. Comes in bra sizes for better fit. Straps can be uncomfortable if not fit properly. Lontex provides a telephone network to answer questions.	Five stars for breathability; three stars for comfort; four stars for support.

*Ratings in three categories: breathability, comfort, and support. Maximum rating five stars.

BRAS FOR LARGER-SIZE WOMEN

Bra	Fabric	Features
Action Shape Sport Top Champion Jogbra	Nylon, Lycra mesh, CoolMax band	Full coverage, especially under the arms to hold large breasts in the bra lines.
Sports Bra, Support Teams	Nylon, Lycra mesh	Nonstretch straps; wide Y back panel provides excellent support.
Sports Top, Champion	Cotton, polyester, Lycra spandex; CoolMax cup liner	Designed for C–DD sizes; clasps in back; support without excess flattening; fits narrow chests.
Comfort-Strap Sport Top, Champion	Cotton, polyester, Lycra; CoolMax liner	Extrawide, cushioned shoulder straps reduce chafing for long runs and high-impact workouts; fits up to DD.
Super Support Underwire Sports Bra, Speedo	Cotton, Lycra	Underwire provides support and nonsport style separation; two-inch-wide band keeps bra in place without chafing or digging; back clasp; wide, adjustable straps.
Underwire Sport Top, Champion	Cotton, polyester; CoolMax mesh liner	Comfortable underwire that provides separation; wires are plush-covered to avoid gouging; pull-over style with back clasp; fits narrow chests.

A BRA-BUYING CHECKLIST

- Before buying a new sports bra, run or walk in what you already own. After the first few days of your program, you'll be able to home in on the features you really need.

- Check the label. It's an excellent source of information. You're looking for a bra made from a breathable, absorbent fabric that wicks heat and sweat away from your body.

- Run your hands along the bra to check that there is no metal or plastic hardware or any raw seams or rough fabric edges that will lie against your skin.

- Feel the fabric. It should be very soft and smooth and a type that resists "pilling" after repeated machine washing and drying. (Fabric that "pills" will chafe.)

- Try on the bra and jump, arms stretched overhead, and jog in place using exaggerated arm and torso movement. The bra should not ride up.

- If the bra survives all these tests, it probably is the right one for you.

WILL WALKING OR RUNNING WITHOUT A BRA CAUSE BREASTS TO SAG?

The simple answers are no and we don't know for sure. But as is the case with many other hot button issues, the answers are never truly that simple. For many years, we were taught that a bra was necessary during exercise to protect our breasts from damage, sagging, and perhaps even breast cancer. Today we realize that many of these warnings reflected mythology rather than fact. Puritanical attitudes that equated unrestricted breasts with unrestricted sexual habits and lingerie advertising that reinforced fears of potential problems resulting from exercising braless formed a powerful combination.

Most sports, including walking, will not damage braless breasts. Many others, such as swimming, weight lifting, yoga, and gymnastics, develop the chest muscles and are breast enhancers. They are also often best performed without a bra. But the jury is still out on high-impact activities such as running, basketball, and jumping rope.

Women with small breasts who usually go braless probably won't notice any difference whether they wear a bra or not. If you have large breasts, which may sag naturally, physics and common sense say running might exacerbate that tendency, and you should find a bra that gives you adequate support.

If you fall somewhere in between, your answer may be determined strictly by your level of comfort. If you have good carriage and muscular development and don't mind a little bouncing when you run, then by all means go without a bra. But if you worry about being conspicuous or feel you need support for your breasts, find one of the comfortable new bra tops and take off.

Whatever bra you choose, you can run with the confidence that this question should not keep you from the sense of accomplishment and the feeling of well-being you can find out on the road.

Like most young women of my generation, I just accepted the fact that a bra was a necessary piece of underwear. If you didn't wear one, your breasts would collapse and sag. Yipes!

During a workout one evening in 1972, after six years of serious running, I suddenly just couldn't stand the chafing across my breastbone anymore. Up until then, I had lived with permanent scarring and scabs on my chest. After long runs, my chest was often raw and bleeding. My shoulders were also badly chafed from metal strap adjusters. I tried to protect myself with tape, gauze pads, and petroleum jelly, all with limited success. At a certain point, friction always wore them off or ruckled them up, and my skin was attacked again.

Besides, the bra wasn't really helping the thing I needed most: controlling the bouncing. Most of the time my running caused me to slip halfway out of the bottom. So I stopped right along the roadside, reached behind, and unsnapped the monster and wriggled out of it. I decided I'd rather have sagging breasts than suffer anymore.

The fact is that most women can't do this. Running without the support of a bra is too painful for them.

A world-class runner friend of mine, now in her forties and still performing at a high level, has the rarest of assets: full, size-B breasts, while the rest of her is absolute skin and bones. (Most world-class runners have such low body fat that they have very small breasts.) My friend has always run with a bra and never more happily than now.

"I love the colorful stretch tops they have now," she says. "I move and breathe freely in them, and they give me enough support. Ten years ago it was terrible trying to find any kind of bra that worked.

"Wearing a bra has always been important for me because I find the flopping extremely distracting to me . . . as well as for others! The few times I ran without a bra, I never heard so many comments or car horns! The flopping *wasn't really uncomfortable, and I was never concerned about breaking down breast tissue because I knew that the strenuous arm movement and deep breathing were also promoting great chest muscle development. The reason a bra was important to me was that it helped my posture. It made me carry myself better. This was important to my running form, and at my level, form is a very important part of performance. I think the guideline here is comfort. Whatever feels all right can't be wrong." I strongly second those thoughts!*

Clothing Do's and Don'ts

- Don't wear bras or panties with lace edges or made mostly of nylon—they will scratch once they get damp. If your underpants are not cotton, make sure they have a cotton crotch, which allows sweat and moisture to be absorbed, reducing the chance of yeast infections. Once you're set with your running or walking program, consider buying underwear made with wicking fabrics, or shorts with attached underpants made with a wicking fabric, to alleviate moisture problems.

- Remove exercise clothes as soon as possible after a workout, particularly damp underwear and shorts. Wear exercise clothes once and wash them as soon as possible afterward. If you wear the clothes without washing them, you are risking fungal infections, skin rashes, pimples on your chest and back, and smelly clothes. If a washing machine is unavailable, scrub key items in a sink or the shower and let them hang dry overnight.

- You almost always need less clothing when you are running or walking than you imagine. The body heats up rapidly, so it is better to wear a little less and feel a bit cool at the start rather than have to take off clothing and carry it. However, tying a wind jacket around your waist if you're feeling warm is convenient and can be handy if a sudden rain appears or the wind picks up, or you start to feel chilled.

- In cold weather, the best way to keep warm is by wearing several light layers of clothing, not by wearing one heavy garment. Warm air gets trapped between the layers and keeps you snug. (See clothing charts, pages 72-75.)

- Some old-fashioned sports gear is still terrific in cold weather because it works on the trapped-air principle. The old baggy sweatsuits made of fuzzy gray cotton keep you in a bubble of warm air. Add tights, a turtleneck, a windbreaker, gloves, and a hat to this trusty suit and you can move around all day in sub-zero temperatures. Oddly, once you get moving, feet seem impervious to cold and usually stay comfortably warm without extra layers of socks, even if you run through icy puddles.

- Most heat is lost through the top of the head, so in cold weather *wear a hat*. In extreme cold and wind, put a hood over the hat. If you can keep the pulse points of the neck and wrists warm, the rest of you will seem fine, too. Gloves that cover the wrists can be taken on and off, and sometimes pulling a long sleeve down over your knuckles is enough to keep you comfortable. Then if it warms up, push up the sleeves.

A personal note:

I still think the best gloves are old gray cotton gardening gloves. You may look like Minnie Mouse out there, but they trap the air, keep your hands very warm, are totally washable, and are great for wiping your nose. I have about ten pairs and wear a clean pair for every run.

Running and Walking Accessories

In the fashion world, accessories are often the extras that make an outfit unique. In sports, accessories are functional items that can make your running or walking safer and more comfortable. They may be simple items you already have or new items you need to buy. Here are some things you absolutely need, others that are optional, and some, such as earphones, that are potentially dangerous.

SUNSCREEN

Essential at any age, and vanity has nothing to do with it. Skin cancer is a reality and is primarily caused by exposure to the sun. When you sunbathe, you're acutely aware of the sun's heat and rays, but when you run or walk, the cooling effect of your own breeze can make you forget that the sun's rays are beating down on you, even in cloudy weather. Put at least a 30 SPF sunscreen on all exposed skin, with extra on your lips. Don't worry, you'll still get some tanning, but it will be safer. (Vanity note: if you crave the athletic look of a tan, do what the babes on *Baywatch* do and get it from self-tanning lotions.)

A personal note:

Most of the many thousands of miles I ran were in the dark because I usually ran at 6 in the morning or after 6 in the evening to accommodate my work schedule. At age forty, my skin looked like I was twenty-five. I thought it was just good genes and good luck.

That same year, I started my own business and was thrilled at last to have my daily run in sunlight. But in two years my face, chest, and arm skin looked ten years older. I was frantic! I thought I had started to age more rapidly, until I realized it was the sun. Now I am a diligent user of sunscreen, even in my cosmetics.

Good luck finding a sunscreen that doesn't sting when it drips down with the sweat on your face into your eyes. For that reason, I wear a hat that completely covers my forehead and wraparound sunglasses. The sunscreen goes on the bottom of my face, neck, and chest whenever I run, as well as on my arms and legs during hot weather.

When you first start using a sunscreen in hot weather, it will make you feel hotter and make your sweat feel oilier and heavier on your body. It's a necessary tradeoff, and eventually you'll get accustomed to the feeling. Store your sunscreen in your shoes or keep it by the door, so you'll never forget it.

SUNGLASSES

Make sure they protect against UV rays. For walking, the kind of sunglasses doesn't make much difference, but for running, you should wear a pair designed for sports. They won't slip down your nose no matter how much you sweat or bounce. Polarized sunglasses are soothing for the eyes and are particularly good if you're exercising on a glaring road surface, in snow-covered areas or, at the other extreme, near a beach. Wraparound style sunglasses not only protect your eyes but also keep harmful sun rays off your vulnerable and easily wrinkled facial skin.

REFLECTIVE GEAR

Many women's schedules force them to run or walk in darkness. In addition to the basic safety tips you need to follow (see Chapter 12), wear clothing with reflective strips that enable you to be seen by motorists, bicyclists, and pedestrians. Most shoes, shorts, pants, and jackets are now made with reflective stripping, but you can add reflective material to clothes you already have, or buy a lightweight reflective vest.

BUM BAG OR FANNY PACK

These small, belted purses are great for long runs or walks. You can carry food and extra clothing, as well as money, keys, and other small necessities.

IDENTIFICATION TAG

Always run or walk with some identification tag showing your name, address, and telephone number, as well as an emergency contact, your blood type, and any allergies you have to medicine. Tie the identification tag to your shoe or carry it in your pocket.

BOTTLE BELT

A belt that lets you carry a bottle of water or energy drink. Originally for cyclists and triathletes, some runners and walkers also carry liquids if they are easily dehydrated and in locations where water is not accessible.

DOG REPELLANT

Peppery solution in a small spray canister that clips on your waistband to repel attacking dogs (and possibly two-legged attackers as well). This is illegal in some locations as it is considered a "weapon." Use as a last resort, as it is highly irritating and may damage a dog's eyes. Few dogs will actually attack you if you face them down (see page 190).

ANTICHAFING PRODUCTS

Petroleum jelly is fabulous in preventing chafing, but it can stain clothes and make them look permanently dirty. It also feels uncomfortable until you get moving. Top runners coat the inside of their thighs, their nipples, and between their toes to cut friction. You may want to put a layer of petroleum jelly on the crotch seams of shorts and the underarm seams of tops, particularly before any very long run or race. Some runners put a strip across their eyebrows to divert the flow of sweat away from the eyes.

A new generation of antichafing products is being introduced. Among those available in some running stores and by mail order are Runner's Lube, Body Glide, SportsSlick, and Sportsloob. Runners who have tested these products agree they are easier to wash off than petroleum jelly and are effective.

EARPHONES

An *absolute no-no* when you are running or walking outdoors! You need to hear what is going around you at all times. Earphones are fine indoors on exercise equipment, such as a treadmill or a step machine. But leave the earphones in the locker if you run on an indoor track. On tight indoor tracks you need to be listening for other runners who may be trying to pass you.

HEART RATE MONITOR

An increasingly popular piece of equipment among athletes who want to exercise at a particular effort level. The monitor is strapped to your chest and keeps track of your exercising heart rate and allows you to keep in your "target zone" consistently.

FIRST AID PRODUCTS FOR RUNNING AND WALKING

There are a wide variety of topical ointments and adhesives designed to handle the abrasions, blisters, and other minor injuries that sometimes accompany workouts.

- *Neosporin* antibiotic ointment is essential for healing open blisters. It now comes in a pain-relief formula containing lidocaine. Carry a tube in your gym bag.

- *New-Skin* is a quick-drying liquid that provides flexible bandagelike protection to cuts, abrasions, and blisters. New-Skin is waterproof and lasts twenty-four to forty-eight hours. It also has an antiseptic to speed healing.

- *Second Skin* moisture pads cool blisters and hot spots on your feet and protect them against rubbing. Adhesive bandages are not effective for runners and walkers because sweating loosens them, so they roll up and create more abrasions and discomfort.

chapter 6

BRAVING MOTHER NATURE

RUNNING AND WALKING IN HOT AND COLD WEATHER

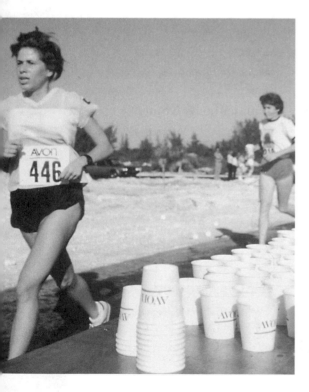

On sultry summer days or when you hear the howling winter winds, it's tempting just to turn over in bed and resolve to wait until fall or spring to run or walk again. But why give up all you've worked so hard to gain just because of the weather? Running and walking are year-round sports. With the right clothing and a few other precautions, you can be as impervious to the elements as the legendary letter carriers have always been.

Keeping Cool in Hot Weather

There is an expression in running that the only thing that can kill you in this sport is heat. Apart from a reckless car, that is mostly true—and a great contrast to most sports where danger, risk, or violence is an inherent part.

What does this expression really mean? When you exercise, you get warm and begin to sweat. Sweat is your body's natural mechanism for cooling: Put wetness on any surface and blow air over it and it becomes cooler. Your body's sweat performs the same function, just as a car radiator does in keeping the engine from overheating.

The danger develops if you overheat and your cooling mechanism doesn't work properly. When that happens, your body temperature spirals upward out of control, and you can suffer heat exhaustion, which can be serious, or much worse, heat stroke, which can be fatal. One of the major causes of heat-related problems for runners and walkers is high humidity. When you sweat in dry air, the air quickly evaporates the moisture and cools you. Humidity prevents rapid evaporation; the moisture stays on the skin, and the body's temperature stays high.

Although some reasons for overheating are beyond your control, most are not. Preparedness and prevention are the best course of action. The following suggestions can help you handle heat.

- **BE GRATEFUL FOR SWEATING.** Beginners, particularly women, sometimes overheat because they do not sweat readily yet—it is as if their body has not yet learned how to completely saturate itself. You see these women all red-faced and puffing away on a warm day but not sweating. Beginners should take everything gradually; when the body acclimates itself to daily exercise, it will begin to sweat on cue. It you are, or become, a copious sweater, be thankful!

- **MAKE WATER YOUR CONSTANT COMPANION.** Drink water all day long—it's hardly ever enough. An important cause of overheating is dehydration, which is the same as not having enough water in your car radiator. Without sufficient water, you don't sweat as much as you need to and therefore don't cool enough.

Another reason for getting lots of water into your system is that blood becomes more "liquid" with a greater volume of fluid in your system. It circulates more easily and moves heat away faster from vital organs.

Stress also dehydrates you, because you are breathing harder and your heart rate becomes elevated. Under stressful conditions, moisture evaporates from your skin and mouth, even when you are not visibly sweating. (This is why you get dry mouth sometimes before speaking in front of a group.) Keep a bottle of water on your desk at work, in a handy place as you move about your house doing chores, or in your car or tote bag when you go out. Drink at least eight large glasses a day. You'll have to urinate more at first, but soon it won't bother you.

When you are exercising you need to really concentrate on taking in enough water. Use gimmicks or tricks to remind yourself to drink enough: Keep a cold water jug in the refrigerator; keep a glass on the kitchen counter; drink one glass when you get up and another every hour; set an alarm during the day if you need to remind yourself!

• **SEVERELY LIMIT YOUR INTAKE OF ALCOHOL WHEN YOU EXERCISE,** particularly in hot weather. Alcohol is very dehydrating, so when you are drinking alcohol, you are losing valuable liquids instead of replacing them. As you run or walk, you're sweating out the already reduced fluids you have, putting more stress on your heart and overheating your system. Alcohol tip: Don't drink *at all* unless you've had a few glasses of water first. Then, with every drink, match it with double the amount of water. You'll feel a lot better the next morning, too!

• **COFFEE, TEA, AND COLAS, FULL OF CAFFEINE, ARE DIURETICS**—substances that promote fluid loss. Match every one of them with a glass of plain water.

Alcohol and exercise can be very tricky. Mixed with heat it can be deadly. One time on a ferociously hot summer day I had a hard workout after work that made me very late for an important reception that evening. I flew into the shower and put on my clothes but neglected to drink a lot of water. When the waiter passed by with a tray of cold champagne, my eyes said "liquid"; I had a glass, quite quickly. And then I had a few more. Never drink alcohol for thirst. Lucky for me, I got sick and took a taxi home even before I became drunk. I could have made a terrible fool of myself. Boy, did I pay. I was deathly ill for two days, worse than any flu I've had. I didn't run well for a week.

GUIDELINES FOR EXERCISING IN HOT WEATHER

- Run or walk during the coolest parts of the day—early morning or early evening.

- Wear light-colored clothing made with the new generation of polyester fabrics, like CoolMax, that are designed to wick the sweat from your skin and cool you. (See Chapter 5 on equipment and clothing.)

- Cotton is still a favorite for T-shirts, but cotton shirts get *very* soggy and hold moisture on your skin, not allowing it to evaporate and cool your body. Wear cotton in more temperate weather.

- Wear as little clothing as possible. Choose loose supplex shorts with a built-in CoolMax panty, a CoolMax crop top, and that's it. Luckily, it is perfectly acceptable for women to wear just shorts and a sports bra. If you feel conspicuous in only shorts and a sports bra, put a loose crop top over the bra. In New York City, women wear the top over the bra while they're going through the streets, but when they hit the park, the top comes off. Tuck it in the back of your shorts, or ball it up and run with it in your hand.

- On hot, humid days, you need to slow down and hose off your body as often as possible. Even though you are covered with greasy-feeling sweat, when you hose down your body with fresh water it keeps you cooler and makes you feel better. Every time you pass someone with a hose, ask him or her to spray you.

- Choose a running route that has water stops. This can be park fountains, spigots outside buildings, neighbors' hoses, or your own—you can do out and back circuits stopping at home for water. Some people go out early and place water bottles along a long route they plan on doing that day. Others have a water bottle-carrying belt, or special shorts with water bottle pockets in the back. (See Chapter 5 on equipment.)

- Wear a white painter's hat that you get in the hardware store and cut lots of holes in it. Fill it with ice as you start your run.

- Totally wet your hair with cold water before you begin your workout.

- Carry a wet washcloth and begin your workout with four ice cubes in it. The cubes will last nearly half an hour. Press the cubes to your face and the back of your neck. Keep the washcloth wet by saturating it with cool water whenever you find it on your running or walking route.

- Wear sunglasses to cut glare.

- Watch out for the following symptoms of heat exhaustion and stop if they occur:
  - feeling dizzy, light-headed, disoriented, nauseated
  - your skin starts to get goose bumps
  - someone says you look pale
  - you suddenly slow down to a crawl for no apparent reason

WHAT TO DO IF YOU OR YOUR RUNNING PARTNER IS SUFFERING FROM OVER-HEATING

Stop running immediately. Get in a cool place, drink as much water as possible, and lie down. Put cool cloths on your body. Immerse yourself in a cool bathtub, if possible. Try to drink some watered-down drink with glucose (sugar) in it—like Gatorade—to bring up your energy a bit. When you feel you can hold food down, eat a banana.

If either of you becomes totally disoriented, or unconscious, call an ambulance. While waiting for it to arrive, put ice on your partner, raising her legs, getting her in air-conditioning, or fanning her like crazy.

A personal note:

On a hot day, after a workout, how do you stop sweating after you get out of the shower? End the shower with a cold rinse. Put your head under the cold water, too. When you get out, dry off standing in front of a fan. Try not to put your clothes on for a while; just put on cotton underpants and a big cotton T-shirt until you settle down. If you have to dress, keep the fan on you and avoid wearing silk, which clings and spots, and settle for linen or cotton.

Cold-Weather Running

A personal note:

Given the choice, I always prefer to run in cold weather rather than hot. Eventually, in cold weather, I can get comfortable if I'm in the right gear. In hot weather, I'm rarely comfortable. I like sweat fine; I just don't like it in my eyes. In the heat, it's always a battle whether I'll be able to finish before the temperature does me in. Afterward, I often feel a little disappointed, probably because I know I'm not moving fast or easily. But in cold weather, I always feel very pure and self-righteous, as if I've conquered the elements.

There are a few drawbacks to running in the cold, namely, that it takes a lot more clothing and more time to get ready. But that's about all. Sure, there are some days when it is really too cold to go out for long workouts. Sometimes there are ice patches that are dangerous, and, with shorter hours of daylight, it's more likely to be dark when you run or walk. But the rest of the time, running or walking in the cold is fabulous. Here are the adjustments you need to keep in mind for maximum comfort and enjoyment.

- **GEAR UP FOR THE DARK.** It will often be dark when you run or walk. Two immediate solutions are: Get a running partner or a coat for your dog. An easier solution may be to run laps in your immediate neighborhood instead of venturing far from home.

- **BECOME A BEACON OF LIGHT IN THE DARK.** Wintertime is often gloomy and overcast, even during the day, so wear bright, reflective gear.

- **WEAR BRIGHT COLORS DURING THE DAY, TOO.** On bright winter days, when you think you are visible, do not wear black pants and gray tops. You'll look exactly like the road and the horizon and be difficult for drivers to see. Go for neon colors.

- **LAYERS EQUAL WARMTH.** During cold weather, it's always better to wear several light layers than one or two heavy garments. Air gets trapped between the layers and keeps you warm. You also feel lighter and more mobile.

- **DON'T OVERDRESS.** When in doubt, leave the extra layer home. You'll be surprised how warm you get running or walking on most cold days. Wear a jacket or windbreaker to keep you warm during the early part of your run or walk, then take it off and tie it around your waist after you're warmed up. It'll come in handy during your cooldown.

- **MOVE INTO** a cold wind for the first part of your run or walk, not away from it. Check the wind direction when you get outside. It is far better to run or walk into the wind at first and then have it behind you coming back. In fact, this is crucial if it is extremely cold and windy outside. If you start your run or walk with the wind behind you, by the time you turn into it on the way back, the wind hitting your already sweaty body will chill you to the bone. Since you are wet and tired, this can, on extreme occasions, cause hypothermia—a potentially dangerous drop in body temperature.

- **BEWARE OF WINDCHILL.** The actual air temperature is usually not the problem in cold-weather running and walking: The windchill factor matters more. Add a stiff wind to cold weather and the temperature feels—and reacts—colder on your body. In cold windy weather, refer to the windchill chart on page 100, make sure you wear a wind jacket and pants over your gear, and finish the workout with the wind at your back. (See Chapter 5 equipment for clothing choices.)

- **PROPER WINTER CLOTHING IS A GOOD INVESTMENT.** This is time to invest in a few key garments, particularly the layer that is closest to your body and your outer shell. You sweat considerably while running and walking in cold weather. Make sure your first layer is made from one of the polyester fabrics that wick off sweat and let it evaporate. What makes you cold is the wet garments against your skin, and it's a miserable feeling. Your outer shell should be made of a breathable, wind-repellent fabric, such as Gore-Tex. You need to get the hot steamy air out but not let the cold winter air blow in. (For more information on clothing selection, see Chapter 5 on equipment.)

- **BUTTON UP TIGHT.** Choose garments that have closures *over* front zippers to keep air and cold rain from leaking through openings and zippers. Getting a jacket and pants that have a snap fold over collar and Velcro closures on the wrist and pants cuffs is worth the investment to keep cold air from rushing down your neck and up the sleeves.

- **DON'T FORGET YOUR HAT AND GLOVES.** Always wear a hat and gloves. You lose a huge amount of body heat right out the top of your head, like a chimney, and through your hands. Look at elite runners in cold weather—they are running in shorts and skinny little singlets but have hats and gloves on.

- **GET OUT OF DAMP CLOTHES AS SOON AS POSSIBLE.** When you stop moving, get out of your workout gear quickly, even if a shower is not in your immediate future. Damp clothing left on the skin chills you very quickly and leaves you feeling miserable for the rest of the day. If you don't plan to go home after a workout or race, take along dry clothes, socks, and a change of shoes; you'll stay comfortable until you can get a hot shower. A hat helps too, particularly if your hair is wet from sweat or rain. In Europe, and increasingly in the United States, people are becoming less shy about whipping off wet clothes after a race and getting into dry gear. Opening a car door and discreetly sitting in the backseat, you can change clothes and no one will notice.

- **HAVE FUN IN THE SNOW BUT BEWARE OF ICE.** Running in fresh snow is one of the most pleasant feelings in the world. Your shoes get a pretty good grip on it, too. When it gets packed, it's still all right for workouts, but you'll go slower. When snow gets icy, find a different route or hit the treadmill. It's not worth the risk of a bad fall to try to run on icy roads. Be particularly careful of black ice, which you cannot see and might mistake for damp spots on the road or sidewalk. Black ice develops first under trees, on bridges, and beside shady banks.

  In really deep snow—knee-deep, for instance—continue walking or jogging. You'll feel like a kid again, and the resistance is very good for you.

• **Help yourself get warm with a stretch.** Always warm up slowly and have a good stretch after you run or walk in the cold. This is more important in the cold than in the heat, because the heat helps you warm up naturally, whereas the cold tightens you. Start your workout more slowly than ever and work into it.

THE HEAT INDEX: HOW HOT IT FEELS

Relative Humidity (%)	Temperature (°F) 70	75	80	85	90	95	100	105	110	115	120
0	64	69	73	78	83	87	91	95	99	103	107
10	65	70	75	80	85	90	95	100	105	111	116
20	66	72	77	82	87	93	99	105	112	120	130
30	67	73	78	84	90	96	104	113	123	135	148
40	68	74	79	86	93	101	110	123	137	151	
50	69	75	81	88	96	107	120	135	150		
60	70	76	82	90	100	114	132	149			
70	70	77	85	93	106	124	144				
80	71	78	86	97	113	136					
90	71	79	88	102	122						
100	72	80	91	108							

At a heat index temperature of:

90–104 Heat cramps or heat exhaustion possible

105–130 Heat cramps or heat exhaustion likely, heatstroke possible

130+ Heatstroke highly likely

Note: Exposure to full sunshine can considerably increase heat index.

WINDCHILL: HOW COLD IT FEELS

Wind (mph)	35	30	25	20	15	10	5	0	-5	-10	-15	-20	-25	-30	-35
5	33	27	21	16	12	7	0	-5	-10	-15	-21	-26	-31	-36	-42
10	22	16	10	3	-3	-9	-15	-22	-27	-34	-40	-46	-52	-58	-64
15	16	9	2	-5	-11	-18	-25	-31	-38	-45	-51	-58	-65	-72	-78
20	12	4	-3	-10	-17	-24	-31	-39	-46	-53	-60	-67	-74	-81	-88
25	8	1	-7	-15	-22	-29	-36	-44	-51	-59	-66	-74	-81	-88	-96
30	6	-2	-10	-18	-25	-33	-41	-49	-56	-64	-71	-79	-86	-93	-101
35	4	-4	-12	-20	-27	-35	-43	-52	-58	-67	-74	-82	-89	-97	-105
40	3	-5	-13	-21	-29	-37	-45	-53	-60	-69	-76	-84	-92	-100	-107
45	2	-6	-14	-22	-30	-38	-46	-54	-62	-70	-78	-85	-93	-102	-109

Actual Temperature (°F)

chapter 7

ALTERNATIVE ROUTES TO SANITY AND VANITY

TREADMILLS, CROSS-COUNTRY SKIING MACHINES, WEIGHT TRAINING, AND HEALTH CLUBS

If you had a dollar for every woman whose running or walking program foundered because of the competing demands for her time, you'd be rich enough to afford the most expensive personal trainer to keep you fit. But for most of us, the reality of too many things to do and too little time to do them needs to be handled on a more practical basis. When you've exhausted all the time management techniques and still can't find

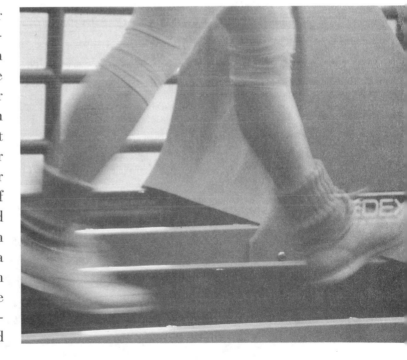

the time to run or walk regularly, the answer may come down to choosing among exercise alternatives.

Your own treadmill or cross-country training machine, weights, a gym, or even a personal trainer to work with you at your gym may offer the flexibility you need to keep your training on schedule, no matter what time constraints you have—and without feeling any guilt over missed runs or walks.

In addition, these alternatives can give variety and balance to your training. An occasional regimen of aerobic classes or swimming at your gym or local Y may be just the tonic to keep you fresh for running or walking. And if you're injured, stationary bikes or swimming can keep your aerobic fitness level up until you recover enough to begin running or walking again.

Finally, most fitness experts now believe that you should try to incorporate balance in an exercise program to achieve total fitness and promote overall well-being. Different activities work different muscle groups to help you achieve maximum flexibility and aerobic capacity while minimizing the possibility of overuse injuries. Select complementary activities—combine running or walking with biking or swimming, for instance—and add strength training to build a program that will keep you fit and enthusiastic.

Let's take a look at some of the best exercise alternatives.

Talking About Treadmills

A personal note:

The treadmill may be the saving of fitness for thousands of women. I've come to this conclusion after nearly fifty thousand beloved miles run in every possible kind of weather and a true hatred of indoor exercise. Treadmills are ugly, expensive, soulless machines that take up a lot of room. But, by heaven, they may be the answer for the truly time challenged and responsibility burdened among us. So if the treadmill fits your lifestyle best, don't look for other answers. Besides, with something that ugly taking up so much of your precious living space, you'll probably use it.

Treadmills are staple pieces of equipment in health clubs and gyms, but here I'm talking about treadmills you purchase for home use. They can be the answer to many time challenges.

- **THE TIME-STRAPPED WORKING WOMAN.** For the working woman who needs to be in the office by 8:00 or 8:30, the treadmill can be a lifesaver. It saves you time in many ways. Instead of dressing for a run, you can roll out of bed and into your sneakers while still wearing whatever you wore for sleeping—that's at least fifteen minutes saved right there. Coiffured hair stays perfect without exposure to wind, rain, or hats, and you're another twenty minutes ahead in hair-washing and blow-drying time. Watch the morning news on television while running or read the newspaper if you walk—twenty more minutes saved. A total of fifty-five minutes on the plus side of the ledger—often the difference between exercising or not.

- **THE MOTHER OR CAREGIVER WHO CAN'T LEAVE HOME TO EXERCISE.** The treadmill enables you to exercise and still keep an eye on those in your care. Moreover, exercise is a great stress reliever, and people confined to a house need a break, even if they can't go out for it.

- **THE WOMAN WHOSE BUSINESS IS IN HER HOME.** Can't afford to miss an important telephone call, fax, or overnight package? Run or walk on your treadmill and you don't have to risk missing anything.

- **THE WOMAN WHO CAN EXERCISE ONLY VERY EARLY IN THE MORNING OR VERY LATE AT NIGHT OR WHO LIVES IN A DANGEROUS NEIGHBORHOOD.** Exercising should always be a stress and tension reducer, so there is no point to exercising in conditions you feel are dangerous. Under any of these circumstances, a home treadmill always fits into your schedule and does so in the safety of your home.

- **THE WOMAN WHO KNOWS SHE WON'T GO OUT TO EXERCISE ONCE SHE'S GOTTEN HOME AT NIGHT.** Whether it's dinner preparation, children, or simply a reluctance to change and go out again, you can easily accommodate exercise to your needs with a home treadmill.

ADVANTAGES AND DISADVANTAGES OF TREADMILL WALKING OR RUNNING

Besides the convenience of an at-home workout, exercising indoors means you don't have to contend with any adverse wind or weather conditions. By regulating the treadmill's speed, you can maintain an exact pace per mile. Or if you want to raise the intensity of your workout, you can increase the incline to make yourself work harder. The machine's surface is also softer and more flexible than most outdoor running surfaces, so it's gentler on your feet and legs.

A personal note:

> Treadmills can put some punch into your workouts. Put yours on an incline so you are working uphill. Adjust the speed of an electric treadmill so you have to move faster. An intensive twenty-minute hill walk will be a lot more useful to you than a twenty-minute saunter. The treadmill can also keep challenging you. Many top athletes use treadmills to get additional work on hills and speed that they may not find outdoors.

The chief disadvantages of a treadmill are cost, space, and monotony. You will probably have to spend from $500 to well over $1,000 on a treadmill, depending on the features you want. Although this is a large outlay of money up-front, you need to weigh it against the treadmill's potential usefulness in helping you maintain your running or walking program over an extended period of time. A good treadmill lasts for many years and yet it costs no more than a one-year gym membership, so over time the high initial cost may turn out to be a real bargain.

Treadmills are large pieces of equipment, and if you live in a small apartment or house it may be out of the question, even if you get the type that folds up. Also, if you put it in the basement or garage to keep it out of sight, it may wind up being out of mind as well, giving you a good excuse to skip a workout.

One of the special joys of running and walking outdoors is the sights and sounds of people and nature you experience. A treadmill can't match that, but it's one piece of exercise equipment for which earphones are ideally suited. You can listen to music, the news, or books on tape (a friend has listened to all of Jane Austen and Charles Dickens on the treadmill). You can set up a television nearby to keep your mind occupied, or place the treadmill near a window or door so you can imagine yourself outside to relieve the tedium.

A personal note:

Ingrid Kristensen, the world record holder in the marathon, had an intense rivalry with Joan Benoit, the United States marathon champion and Olympic gold medalist. During the height of their competition against each other, Ingrid, who lives in Norway, trained indoors on a treadmill during the winter facing a big poster of Joan Benoit.

SETTING UP AN EXERCISE ROUTINE FOR THE TREADMILL

To get the maximum benefit of running or walking on a treadmill, you need to establish the proper pace. You can easily adjust the speed of the treadmill and walk faster to keep up that pace, but if it is too fast for you, there is a risk of injury. Dr. Ayne Furman, who has seen an increase in treadmill-walking injuries, suggests that you establish a baseline pace by determining your running or walking pace on a mile track (or a mile course on the streets you normally use) and then set the treadmill to that time. You can gradually increase the pace, just as you would for outdoor running or walking, but only as you feel yourself gaining strength and stamina. Don't set the treadmill faster and strain to keep up with an unrealistic pace.

Cross-Country Skiing Machines

These machines simulate outdoor cross-country skiing, one of the best forms of aerobic exercise. The cardio-vascular benefits of cross-country skiing, running and walking are very similar, and many well-known marathon runners, including nine-time New York City Marathon champion Grete Waitz, are former cross-country skiers.

A cross-country skiing machine has the additional feature of allowing you to vigorously exercise your upper body. These machines are not powered by electricity. The training effect results from sliding your feet forward and back, while your hands also pull up and back, as if you were using poles in cross-country skiing. Once you become proficient with these machines, they provide an excellent overall workout with little stress on your feet and legs.

The most widely known and popular cross-country skiing machines are manufactured by NordicTrack and are available at stores across the country. They cost between $500 and $800.

Weights and Weight Training

Weights are not an essential part of an effective running or walking program, but they can be an invaluable aid in your quest for overall physical well-being. Running or walking will transform your body, but weight training can speed up the process of reclaiming lost skin tone and elasticity, increase strength and flexibility, and build muscle—all keys to helping your body resist the tendency to gain fat as you age.

Research has shown that as you get older (the process may begin as early as age thirty), you begin to lose muscle mass. Rebuilding muscle mass is one way of speeding the rate of your metabolism, which leads to the burning of more calories during exercise and a reduction in the buildup of fat.

Finally, and perhaps most important for women over the age of forty, the weight-bearing exercises you do as part of a weight-training program contribute to the buildup and maintenance of bone mass, a further deterrent against osteoporosis.

No matter what your age, it's not too late—or too early—to start a weight training program. The following exercises are a basic weight-training program that you can do at home with minimum of equipment—a couple of weights, a towel or mat for floor exercises—and maximum benefit.

UPPER ARMS—BICEPS AND TRICEPS

Start with two-, three-, or five-pound weights depending on your fitness level. Do sets ten repetitions with a minute rest between each set. Aim to do three sets for the biceps and four sets for the triceps.

Biceps curl

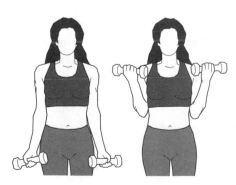

Stand with your feet together and back straight. Hold your arms straight down, next to your body, with your elbows close to your waist. Grip the weights in the palms of your hands, facing forward.

Slowly raise the weights until they reach shoulder level, keeping your elbows close to your waist. Then slowly return to your original position. Don't touch your shoulders with the weights.

Inhale as you lower the weights, exhale as you raise them.

Biceps hammer curl

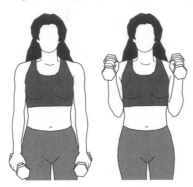

Stand with back straight, feet together, knees slightly bent, and stomach tucked in. This time hold your arms with the weights in your palms facing down.

Slowly raise the weights to your shoulders. Then slowly bring arms down to starting position.

Overhead triceps extension, lying down

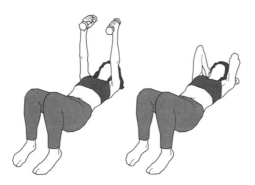

Lie on the floor, with back flat, knees bent, feet on the floor. Extend arms and weights straight overhead with palms facing each other.

Keeping your elbows and upper part of your arms stationary, slowly lower your forearms to your ears. Slowly return forearms to their original position.

Keep elbows in line with your shoulders throughout the exercise.

Triceps kickbacks

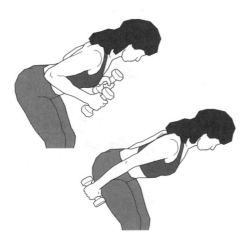

Stand with knees slightly bent. Bend at the waist, with your back straight to a forty-five-degree angle. Keep elbows bent, near to your body.

Slowly extend your forearms backward, wrists stiff and upper arms quiet and in place. Slowly return arms to their original position.

LEGS AND BUTTOCKS

Lunges are terrific for working your thighs, buttocks, and hamstrings. For the novice, the biggest challenge can be keeping your balance. Take a *big* step forward. At first it probably will be easier to do, say, ten lunges with one foot, then ten with the other. When you become more accomplished, alternate right, left, right, left.

Dumbbell lunge

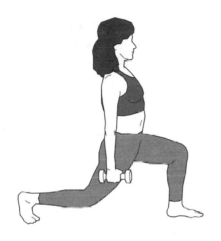

Stand with feet together, back straight, stomach muscles contracted, chest and shoulders high and relaxed. Hold dumbbells straight down at your sides, palms facing in.

Step forward with your right leg until your thigh is almost parallel to the floor. Bend your lower rear knee but don't hit floor. Return to starting position and repeat.

Form is important to this exercise, so try it without weights until you are comfortable. Toes should always point forward. Keep the knee of the forward leg above the ankle—not in front of it— during the lunge and hips from falling below the knee line.

ARMS, SHOULDERS, AND CHEST

For some reason, women *hate* push-ups. At first, they are hard. But the good news is that you see improvement very quickly. One day you can do two push-ups, two days later you can do five. After a month you can do twenty. This is very heartening.

The traditional push-up is one of the best fundamental strengthening exercises. But for many beginners it may place too much strain on the lower back, so start by trying the modified push-up. They do the same job—and eventually you can try the full push-up. Begin with three sets of five, then increase the number and sets. Tip: widen your hands to work your chest muscles more.

If you have problems with your wrists or elbows, you can do a variation. Lie on your back, with legs bent. With your upper arms straight out perpendicular to your body, and forearms pointing to the ceiling, raise hand weights until your arms are straight. Lower your arms to just above the floor (try not to rest your arms between reps). Repeat until you are really tired, as these aren't as effective as actual push-ups.

Traditional push-up

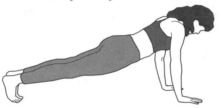

Lie with your body off the floor resting on toes and hands, arms straight and shoulder width apart, fingertips forward.

Slowly, lower your body straight down, without touching the floor, and then slowly push yourself up to the starting position. Keep back and buttocks flat.

Bent knee push-up

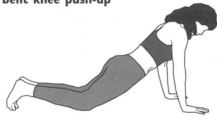

Kneel on hands and knees with legs crossed in back. Place hands shoulder width apart, fingertips facing forward, arms straight. Contract stomach.

Lower your chest until you are just about to hit the floor, then push upward to your starting position.

TIP

"Negative only" exercises are perfect for women—such as new mothers—who don't have enough strength to do regular exercises yet. For instance, when doing sit-ups, just lower yourself down from a sitting position, push yourself up with your hands and lower yourself down again—it's the same muscle group. For push-ups, lower yourself slowly to the floor, relax, roll over, and start from the top again.

ABDOMINALS

These abdominal exercises strengthen your stomach muscles without straining your back. Do the abdominal curl first, then add the others to your workout. Start with five to ten repetitions. Remember: Keep your lower back flat on the floor during all of these exercises.

Abdominal curl

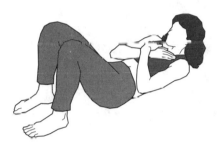

Lie on your back with knees bent, feet flat and hands across your chest. Keep your back flat to the floor throughout the exercise.

As you exhale, curl up, bringing your shoulders off the floor. Keep your head still and your chin close to your chest. Lower yourself to the floor, so that your shoulders touch, but the back of your head does not quite reach the floor.

Repeat at medium speed, building a rhythm in your movement. Tip: Lift yourself up by your abdominal muscles, don't jerk upward with your head and shoulders.

Elbow-knee ab curl

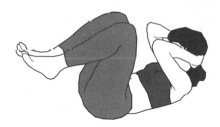

Start in the same position as for the abdominal curl. Lace your fingers behind your head, at ear level, and using your abdominal muscles raise yourself from the floor. Raise your feet up off the floor.

Move your elbows and knees toward each other, stopping with your elbows about an inch or two from your knees. Uncurl and then repeat. Be careful not to pull or strain your neck!

Alternating elbow-knee ab curl

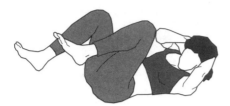

Use the same starting position for the elbow-knee ab curl. With your shoulders raised off the floor, alternate touching your right elbow to left knee and then left elbow to right knee. Touch each knee for one count. To get the most out of the exercise, move your knees straight forward and back, like riding a bicycle, and turn your body slightly from side to side to touch your knees.

A personal note:

I keep a couple of substantial soup cans stashed under the living room sofa and use then as weights while I watch the evening news. When I get more ambitious, I use free weights I have set up in the garage. I bought this set— bar, weights, props, and bench—at a yard sale for $75. Yard sales almost always have weight sets for sale because people buy with the best of intentions and then don't use them. Don't make the same mistake.

TIP

Abdominal crunches are a real powerhouse for runners and walkers. Many back injuries are caused by weak abdominal muscles, a major area of concern for women over forty. Unfortunately, running and walking won't strengthen your abs, so sit-ups are important. Not only do they help prevent injury but they flatten your tummy as well.

Health Clubs and Gyms

For women under forty, physical fitness has emerged as a new standard of beauty to an unprecedented degree. The stars of the entertainment and fashion worlds are lean, with a sleek, well-toned look. They are working out, and younger women are following their lead. Nothing symbolizes this change more than the health club business. It's booming as women use the clubs as multipurpose fitness and social centers. Unfortunately, this view of reality is often reversed for many women over forty. They often see health clubs as sophisticated gyms, where men and unfamiliar equipment traditionally reign supreme.

In truth, health clubs are wonderful for some women and intensely depressing to others. Women with exercise experience often find health clubs a great place to go to work out regularly or as an addition to a running or walking program. They provide a variety of exercise alternatives—from treadmills and stationary bicycles to aerobic classes, pools, and weight-training equipment—and a fully equipped locker room for showering and dressing is open early in the morning and late at night. Many clubs offer extras such as sauna, massage, a snack and juice bar, and child care. Men and women often use the club as a social gathering place, where you can meet friends for a class or just enjoy working out in a social atmosphere.

As wonderful as a club membership can be, it does come at a price measured financially and in terms of convenience and comfort. For a woman with no fitness experience, the idea of even walking into a gym for the first time is intimidating. While health clubs are filled with people of all ages and shapes, to a fifty-five-year-old woman, for example, who has never done any exercise before, every person in the club looks like a Lycra-clad sylph. Overall, two thirds of people who join health clubs never come back. Before joining a club, you have to ask yourself what you really want from it and what you can actually expect to receive. And then use it!

HEALTH CLUB CHECKLIST

- Gym memberships are expensive, and most people think they've purchased fitness when they join. In truth, they have bought only the facility in which to *work on* fitness.

- Exercising in a health club is more time-consuming than doing it on your own. You have to add at least thirty minutes to your workout to account for travel time to the club, changing, showering, and going back home. Since lack of time is the single biggest barrier to a woman maintaining an exercise program, this extra time can mean the difference between working out or not. In thirty minutes you can complete a great workout at your house. If you decide to join a club, get the most convenient one possible.

- Health clubs have a tendency to be most crowded just when you want to be there. Waiting for a piece of equipment wastes time and may eventually deter you from going at all. Try using waiting time to strike up new friendships or scheduling some workouts before or after peak periods.

- While some women like having other people around them when they exercise, others like privacy during a workout. It is a time for yourself and you don't want to feel self-conscious about your jiggling thighs, lack of makeup or ragged gym clothes. It's not possible to be totally anonymous in a club, but the truth is that no one really cares. However, if you *think* people are looking at you and that makes you uncomfortable, a health club may not be for you.

- If you've never gone to a gym before, take advantage of the trial memberships most gyms offer. Use it for a week and see if you like the experience. Also try to get a friend to join with you. The two of you can go for workouts together until you're ready to go it alone.

- Personal trainers are also available at clubs. They work with you until you feel comfortable with the club and its equipment and, for a fee, can become your personal instructor and help you stay motivated until you can do it for yourself.

chapter 8

MANAGING YOUR TIME

YOU REALLY *DO* HAVE TIME TO EXERCISE

A personal note:

Guilt is a big part of the reason women don't run or walk. We feel guilty about taking time for it and we feel guilty if we don't take the time. I finally decided I was not going to feel guilty about running. That thirty minutes to one hour a day I spend running is not only the most important hour of the day, it's the best. Running has given me everything—my career, my husband, my sense of self. The minute I start to think that I should do some more work— when it's already well after six or seven o'clock— and skip my running, I tell myself that's crazy, and I hit the road.

Time is perhaps the greatest gift and cruelest curse of our lives. We worry about how to use it wisely. We try to save it. We see it moving too quickly. And we *very* often feel we don't have

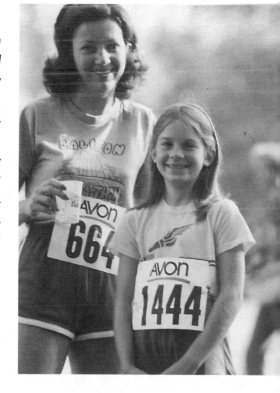

enough of it. Running and walking can sometimes feel like just one more item to add to your list of things to do.

Time is an important issue for all women, particularly for a woman over forty. Turning forty is one of life's major markers. It means we are at the threshold of middle age and, on many levels, it's the beginning of a long series of transitions to come.

For many women, it's a time to evaluate your place in the world and your connection to those things most important to you. Work, family, and relationships may be in a state of flux as you get older.

Whether you are new to the workplace or have always balanced a career with a more traditional woman's role, your forties introduces a period of intense job obligations and potential rewards. You may be just hitting your professional stride. Or if you are beginning a career or have recently returned to the workplace, you face pressure to prove your capabilities.

At the same time, family responsibilities remain constant. If you had children in your twenties, now they are teenagers whose needs are still an important consideration in allocating your time. For those who delayed childbearing, there are young children needing your attention. You may also be a key caregiver for elderly parents, who are living longer and need your assistance in handling the demands of their lives.

And let's not forget romance. Married, single, or divorced, relationships require time and attention, just like everything else in your life.

When you were younger, it seemed you could juggle all of these roles—plus others—more easily. If you had to get a little less sleep one night, you'd make up for it the next. Today, experts who study sleeping and its role in our health agree that we need about eight hours a night. If you "lose" sleep during the week, you can't make it up by sleeping later on weekends.

Everyone needs regular rest. As you get older, it becomes an even greater issue. Sleep patterns change, so it is sometimes more difficult to get to sleep and to sleep deeply through the night. The onset of menopause is often marked by broken sleep. Fortunately, regular exercise is a lifesaver in promoting sound sleep.

So how can you fit running or walking into your busy life? You can't expand the hours in a day, but you can change how you view time and the priorities you set for various activities. Just like an investor in the stock market who's looking for the greatest return on his or her money, exercise is an investment of time and effort that can be judged by its return on assets spent. It is an investment in *yourself*.

Running and Walking: Indulgence or Investment?

A personal note:

In 1977, I stopped running competitively and began to channel that energy into my career. At the time, I was commuting from a suburb north of New York City to a job in Manhattan, a couple of wasted hours a day. I decided to move into Manhattan and take an apartment that allowed me to walk to work. The rent was enormous by the standards of the time, but I looked on it as an investment in myself and my future. Living just a few blocks from the office meant I could get in earlier, work later, and get in several runs a week. My career took off as I found myself better organized and more rested than I had been in my commuting days. And I got fit again. It was an investment that paid huge dividends.

Webster's dictionary defines *indulgence* as the gratification of a desire, while it describes *investment* as using time, talent, and emotional energy to achieve something. That's a nearly perfect description of what it takes to begin and maintain a running or walking program. So if you're feeling the least bit selfish about taking a run or walk before performing some chore at home, keep this definition in mind. What you are doing is not an indulgence but an investment—even though you will get a lot of pleasure out of your workout.

Running and walking programs offer immediate and long-term benefits for the investment of time you put into them. You will look and feel better. You'll have more strength and stamina and feel less stressed.

If you've fought throughout your life to manage your weight, exercise will give you a way to seize the upper hand in that battle once and for all. It can liberate your mind from the cycle of hunger and negative body image and your pocketbook from the expense of diet books and diet foods. Walking and running give you a realistic way of achieving your goals.

Running and walking also provide you with some private time. You can use this space to reflect on the day's events, think through a problem, or just let your mind wander, while enjoying the feeling of movement itself.

If you run or walk with a partner or group, you can enjoy the camaraderie that comes from accomplishing shared goals and having fun.

But first you need to believe you deserve it. Yes, it's something you are doing for yourself. And yes, you will need to take time from something—or someone—else to accomplish it. But don't be sidetracked by guilt. If you don't do it for yourself, who will do it for you?

A personal note:

Letting my mind free-float during a walk or run is therapeutic for me; it's another form of dreaming. The demons come out, the creative comes in.

Running and Walking: Making It a Priority

A basic tenet of time management is to establish priorities. First you decide what's important, then you establish where to place a particular activity or project on your to-do list. Very often when we say we don't have time to do something, it means we don't see that activity as a priority. This is especially true for women and exercise. We make time for those things that are important to us, so you need to decide how important running or walking is to you.

If running or walking becomes one of your must-do activities, then you'll start to look at how you can create the time for it on your daily schedule. Rather than taking the time from just one place by totally eliminating something else, try to find ways to slice a little time from several things, until you have another thirty to thirty-five minutes during the day.

For example, one place to start may be meal preparation. Since it's quicker to heat something frozen than to cook it from scratch, you may want to spend time on the weekend cooking and freezing meals for the following week. There are opportunities like this throughout your daily activities, like the time and method you take to dress, shop, do hair and makeup, and make phone calls. Review everything for time efficiency and you'll find your commitment time.

Get Full Value for the Time You Devote to Exercise

Look at time as a gift, even if it is only five, ten, or fifteen minutes, and do everything you can to make it work for you.

Running or walking are ideal exercises for many reasons, not the least of which is how much they give back in terms of time invested. If you choose swimming as your cardiovascular workout, you have to add time going to and from the pool, then changing and drying off to your basic thirty-minute workout. You may spend twice your actual workout time nonproductively, a heavy burden to add to your already difficult schedule. On the other hand, thirty minutes spent running or walking give you just that amount of exercise. If you add fifteen minutes for cooling down and stretching, that's forty-five minutes of productive time. Almost every moment you put into running or walking produces some training benefit.

In addition, running and walking can be done almost anywhere and at virtually any time. If you drive a lot, keep an extra pair of sneakers, a towel, a water bottle, and a change of clothes in your car so you're always ready to take advantage if an unexpected opportunity for a workout develops. Perhaps your last appointment of the day cancels. Now you have a free thirty minutes. If you have that full gym bag in the car, you can be out running or walking, or at the gym, without having to go home and get your things.

Be imaginative about carving out time for exercise in your everyday schedule. For example, although thirty to thirty-five minutes of running or walking three or four times a week is your goal, you don't have to do it all at once. If you have ten or fifteen minutes of free time before your children get home, use it for a run or walk, either outdoors or on a treadmill. Then you can do the rest of your workout later.

Become More Time Efficient

Exercise not only makes you more aware of time, it also can teach you how to use it more efficiently. In order to accommodate your commitment to running or walking, you're going to need to be more resourceful in organizing your time.

There are two keys: Plan ahead and pay attention to details. For instance, if you run or walk in the morning, lay out your clothes the night before; do it before you leave for work if you run right after you get home.

Other ways to plan ahead and save time:

- Put your shoes, keys, pocket change, and any other small items you need next to the door, so you don't forget anything your need and have to come back once you've started your workout.
- Buy enough socks, shorts, and T-shirts so that no matter how infrequently you do laundry, you always have clean clothes to wear.
- Avoid duplication of effort. Plan workouts for when you won't have to redo hair and makeup after you shower.

Make everything associated with your workout as routine as possible. If you think out the details in advance, you'll spend less time preparing and more time getting on with your program.

Soon the good habits you develop to accomplish your workouts will become a part of your everyday life. You'll be more organized and efficient in your use of time. And that will make time seem more like a friend than an enemy.

A personal note:

I talk to a lot of women who exclaim, "Go for a run or walk? Are you crazy? I don't have the time!" Yet they have time to walk around the mall for an hour. What these women don't realize is that there is time to run or walk, if they manage their time better.

Make Running and Walking Part of Your Routine

You wouldn't walk out of the door without showering, brushing your teeth, or combing your hair, would you? Well, perhaps to pick up the mail or the morning newspaper. But otherwise, those things make up your daily routine. Each person has many others, as well. Taking your vitamins, a telephone call to children or parents, a check of the dog or cat's water dish.

What's routine? It's those things you do without needing to think "is this a necessity?" or "is this important?" Running and walking should join that list. When you make it part of your routine, family, friends, and coworkers will recognize and respect your commitment. They'll also be less likely to interfere with your workout time because they know how important it is to you.

The time of day you exercise is a matter of personal choice. You may need to begin the day with exercise to get yourself going, or you may prefer to work out at night to leave behind the stresses and demands of the day. And, of course, you have to be flexible. Other demands may make a morning run necessary even though you're an evening exercise person or force you to skip a day. Keep in mind that it's more important that you run or walk at all than that you do it at a particular time. A change in routine can be refreshing. And if you miss a day, just make sure to get back to your program as soon as you can.

When the day feels incomplete without a run or walk, it means you've crossed a psychological barrier. Exercise is now a part of your life. It's something you look forward to and need. And it's something that will be there for you through the rest of your life.

Take heart in your quest to fit running or walking into your busy life. Every woman you see on the road, going into a gym, or power walking around your block has faced the same dilemma and overcome it. You can too! There's no need to reinvent the wheel. These tips have worked for other women and will for you.

Time Management Tips

FOR ALL RUNNERS OR WALKERS:

- Find a running or walking partner. A partner can be a godsend in terms of time management. Agree on a time and place to meet and that if either is five minutes late, the other is free to start. The commitment is there, but no one has to be keep waiting too long. If you miss each other one day, you can just meet for your next scheduled run.

     Partners provide motivation, safety, companionship. It's nice to share your achievements and work toward a goal together. And if you're new to athletics, you can provide each other moral support as you venture out into this new world.

- Want a partner but don't know anyone who wants to join with you? Check with your local running or walking club. The New York Road Runners Club has a "matching service"—in many ways it's also a type of matchmaking service—that helps runners find partners of similar pace to run with at various times of the day. Some Ys and community centers have groups and partner services. If your local club doesn't have this kind of program, suggest that it start one.

- Turn chores into running or walking opportunities. If you need to go to the post office or the library, run or walk instead of taking your car. You can do the same thing for any number of small chores. Wear a running or walking backpack and you'll have room for books or small purchases. If your dog trots along beside you, you don't have to take him or her for a separate walk.

- Join the predawn walking group at the mall and case the windows to speed shopping later.

- If all else fails, think about purchasing a treadmill. A treadmill in your bedroom, recreation room, or basement can be the ultimate time-saving piece of equipment. It's right there, all the time, waiting for you. (For details on the advantages and disadvantages of treadmills, see Chapter 7 on equipment.)

For mothers with Children:

- Take preteens or teenagers along on your workout. By making your run or walk a family activity, not only will you ensure that your kids are engaging in a healthful activity but you also get some quality time together. They can bike or roller blade alongside, too. And don't you wish someone had gotten you into the habit of exercising twenty-five years ago?

- Share child watching with your exercise partners. If you all have small children, make up a schedule that rotates child-watching chores evenly so no one misses consecutive workouts.

- Consider buying a baby jogger. Kids love being a part of your run or walk, and once your child outgrows it, you can pass the baby jogger along to a friend or relative.

- Make deals with neighbors. If your close neighbor doesn't have kids or like to run or walk, she can still be of help. Arrange a tradeoff—if she watches your child while you run, then you can pick up groceries or wait for a delivery or repairperson for her.

- Take your children along to the high school track. While you run laps, they can play on the infield where you can easily keep an eye on them.

- Does your husband or partner run or walk? Arrange complementary workout schedules, so each of you can exercise and watch your children.

For working women:

All of the preceding ideas apply to you, but since you are already out of the house and on an imposed schedule—your boss's—you have other opportunities.

- Do your workout on the way home. Whether you have a family or are single, going out again after you get home is very difficult. However, if you bring your workout clothes and a towel with you in the morning, you can get in a run or walk before you get home.

  Change in the bathroom at work, then either establish a route right from the office door or drive to a favorite path or track. After your cooldown, you can drive home in your warm-up suit.

  Train, bus, or subway commuters can do virtually the same thing. You may want to run or walk near your office and pick up your clothes after your workout. Or if you leave your car at the train or bus station, drop off your clothes in it and drive to your favorite running or walking route.

- Use flextime to create a convenient workout schedule. Today, many businesses offer flextime schedules. Whether you like to exercise early or late, this type of schedule can give you the flexibility you need to balance other responsibilities with running or walking.

- Start a running or walking group at work. If you would feel conspicuous going out of your office in running or walking clothes, use your company newsletter or bulletin boards to find other women who also want to workout at work. There is safety and anonymity in numbers, and you'll probably find many like-minded coworkers. And they don't have to all be women!

- Business travelers: Running or walking is a great way to see some of the cities you visit outside the confines of a conference room. Most hotels now provide walking/running maps. Or pre-outline a route to take in some of the location's top sights. Go out early, as meetings often stretch into dinner.

- Conventions almost always have a "happy hour" from 5 to 7. Steal away and exercise during this time, appearing back fifteen minutes before it's over. Inevitably, it's just in full swing! Caution: don't drink alcohol until you've had *plenty* of water!

The battle with time is a fight we have all our lives. Don't feel discouraged by it. One characteristic of runners and walkers is their ability to get on with the task at hand. If you believe in what you are doing and the results you'll achieve, then the rest will fall into place. Please share your time management tips. They'll help someone else find out that running and walking are the fast track to looking good and feeling better—just as you did.

chapter 9

EATING AND EXERCISE

THE NUTRITIONAL COMPONENT OF SANITY AND VANITY

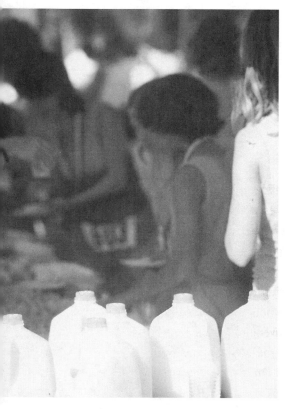

A personal note:

I used to think it was important to keep my weight down, so I cut back on food, forgetting that food is fuel and I needed to eat enough to train hard. Tired and depressed, I didn't run well.

I found that when I ate more I could keep my energy up and really train hard. Then weight just fell off me. Best of all, I felt wonderful, and my running really improved. It took me years to figure this out. I wish I had known this in my twenties.

For women, there is almost no subject as bound up in myth and conflicted feelings as eating. Who would want to forgo the pleasure of eating a wonderful, tasty meal, savoring every bite and walking away from the table full and satisfied? Of course, no one would. But for women it's not that easy.

For most of us, food exists as much as a symbol of how we feel about ourselves as it does for what it really is: the fuel that powers our bodies. Too often we board the merry-go-round of weight gain, dieting, self-recrimination, and more dieting. Food becomes the enemy, and poor eating habits result. Our concern centers on how much we weigh and what size clothing we wear rather than how energetic, healthy, and content we feel.

However, there are also legitimate worries about the effect of fat, cholesterol, and food additives on heart disease, cancer, osteoporosis, obesity, and other illnesses. It's no wonder the subject of food and nutrition causes such frustration and confusion.

It doesn't have to be this way. By choosing to run or walk, you've opened a door to a new way of living where healthful eating and weight control are part of an overall approach to physical and mental well-being. Exercise and proper eating are intertwined. A balanced diet gives you the energy you need to run or walk, while exercise burns calories and fat to help you control your weight with more success than you may have ever had before.

Exercise alone is not a miracle diet plan. But combine it with proper nutrition, and you're on your way to a healthier lifestyle.

A personal note:

Too many women see themselves as somehow deficient because they don't look as good or aren't as thin as the media images we're bombarded with. Even among otherwise very successful women, self-esteem is often very low, due to negative body image: Preoccupied with weight and aging, they feel victims of their own bodies. The first line of defense here is to get positive: Actively do something! Walking and running are perfect—they are accessible, fun, and effective. The next is seriously to address your own body image: Why are you conforming to someone else's standards of attractiveness? You deserve to be happy now, and part of that is acceptance of what you are now, what you are doing now, not what you will be "someday . . . when I'm thin." Strive for health and movement, and all else will follow.

The Keys to a Healthful Diet

Throughout our lives we've been getting instruction on what we should eat to stay healthy. All the mothers and grandmothers who told us to eat a good breakfast, finish our vegetables, and keep away from sweets had the right idea all along. In 1990, the U.S. Department of Agriculture (USDA) published dietary guidelines that Mom probably had a hand in writing, so closely did they mirror her admonitions.

The guidelines recommend: Eat a variety of food; choose a diet low in fat, saturated fat, and cholesterol and high in vegetables, fruits, and grains; restrict the use of sugar and salt; and drink alcoholic beverages in moderation.

In fact, the USDA took the guidelines one step farther, illustrating them in a pyramid that shows how to build a balanced diet.

Choosing from these food groups, you can eat a varied diet. And in food, variety is not only the spice of life, it ensures that you get all the nutrients you need to keep you strong and healthy.

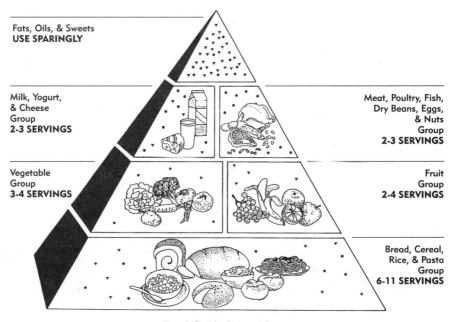

Fats, Oils, & Sweets
USE SPARINGLY

Milk, Yogurt,
& Cheese
Group
2-3 SERVINGS

Meat, Poultry, Fish,
Dry Beans, Eggs,
& Nuts
Group
2-3 SERVINGS

Vegetable
Group
3-4 SERVINGS

Fruit
Group
2-4 SERVINGS

Bread, Cereal,
Rice, & Pasta
Group
6-11 SERVINGS

Food Guide Pyramid

THE SIX BASIC NUTRIENTS

Carbohydrates	Fruits, vegetables, breads, and grains are the primary source of the energy you need to exercise. They provide calories from sugars and starches.
Fat	Source of energy for long-term activity. Choose vegetable fats that are generally unsaturated and less harmful, such as olive oil, corn oil, and canola oil.
Protein	Protein is essential when you exercise. It builds and repairs muscles and reduces the risk of iron deficiency and anemia. Choose among fish, poultry, lean meat, beans, soy, and legumes. You need sufficient protein, and you can find low-fat alternatives to traditional red beef.
Vitamins	Vitamins control chemical reactions in your body. Essential vitamins include A, B complex, C, D, E, and K. Your body does not produce vitamins; you must get them from the food you eat.
Minerals	Calcium, iron, potassium, and sodium are some of the key minerals your body requires. Like vitamins, your body does not produce minerals; you must get them from food.
Water	Water makes up approximately 60 to 75 percent of your weight. It carries nutrients to cells, helps regulate body temperature, and eliminates waste from cells.

Putting Together a Healthful Diet

Nancy Clark, a leading sports nutritionist, describes three keys to healthful eating:

- *Variety:* There isn't one magic food. Each food offers you different and necessary nutrients, so make sure you don't become too attached to one personal favorite or you might be short-circuiting your overall diet.

- *Moderation:* Even soda and chips, in moderation, can fit into a well-balanced diet. The secret: Balance out refined sugars and fats with nutrient-wise choices at your next meal. Although, no one food is a junk food, too many nutrient-empty choices can evolve into a junk food diet.

- *Wholesomeness:* Choose natural or lightly processed foods as often as possible. For instance, whole wheat rather than white bread, apples instead of apple juice, or a baked potato instead of French fries. Natural foods usually have more nutritional value and fewer questionable additives.

The next step is putting this information together with specific foods to develop your own healthful and satisfying diet. You have a lot of choices, so you can balance good nutrition with interesting and tasty food. This is not a diet in the traditional sense, a list of things you *can't* eat that feels like punishment. Instead, it's a wide variety of foods you *can* eat and enjoy.

BREAD, CEREAL, RICE, AND PASTA

All of these are important sources of carbohydrates, fiber, and B vitamins. Grains and starches energize muscles, protect against muscle fatigue, and increase bowel regularity, and they are naturally low in fat and calories. The best choices are lightly processed breads and grains, such as whole wheat bread, brown rice, and stoned wheat crackers. The list is not narrow: bagels; whole wheat, rye, or pumpernickel breads; bran and oat bran cereals; low-fat muffins are there for starters.

FRUITS AND VEGETABLES

Fruits and vegetables provide vitamins C and A, potassium, carbohydrates, and fiber. These nutrients can improve healing, reduce the risk of cancer and high blood pressure, and relieve constipation. They also aid in recovery after exercise.

There is great interest in the health properties of the antioxidant nutrients found in vegetables. These nutrients include vitamin C, carotenoids, vitamin E, and some minerals. Scientists believe they are potentially beneficial in reducing the risk of cancer and certain chronic diseases.

Among the best **fruit** choices you can make are citrus fruits, such as oranges, grapefruits, and tangerines. Although whole fruits have slightly more nutritional value, fruit juices are a good on the go alternative. Look for true fruit juices, not "juice drinks" that have small amounts of juice and a lot of sugar and artificial flavoring.

It seems that nature invented the banana with athletes in mind. Bananas are low in fat and high in fiber and potassium, and they come neatly packaged to go anywhere your walking and running take you. They are a natural energy booster and can be combined with such other foods as cereals, yogurt, crackers, and peanut butter for a nutritious meal.

Among other nutritionally potent fruits are cantaloupe, kiwi, strawberries and dried fruits.

Vegetables are chock full of vitamins you need. Vitamin C and beta- and other carotenes, potassium, and magnesium just scratch the surface of the nutritional benefits you'll get from eating sufficient quantities of vegetables.

In general, darker, more colorful vegetables contain more nutrients than paler ones. Put broccoli, spinach, green peppers, tomatoes, and carrots ahead of mushrooms, cucumbers, and pale lettuces.

Don't forget the cabbage family—cabbage, cauliflower, brussels sprouts, bok choy, collards, and kale. These vegetables are rich in nutritional value and may protect against cancer. The same is true for carotene-rich vegetables such as carrots, winter squash, and greens.

FRESH, FROZEN OR CANNED— WHAT'S THE BEST VEGETABLE CHOICE?

Although fresh vegetables are always the preferred choice because they are nutritional powerhouses, if convenience and price are key considerations, canned or frozen vegetables shouldn't be ignored. There is little nutritional difference between canned and frozen vegetables, and both provide a good percentage of the nutrients you need from the vegetable group. Overcooking vegetables, in whatever form you buy them, is the real killer of nutritional value. So don't leave vegetables off your table because your favorites are out of season or not available in the fresh produce section. Check the shelves or freezer, and you'll probably find what you want there.

MILK, YOGURT, AND CHEESE

Dairy products supply your body with calcium, protein, and riboflavin. They help you maintain strong bones, reduce the risk of osteoporosis, and protect against high blood pressure and muscle cramps. You can maintain a low-fat diet and still get sufficient dairy products by choosing low-fat milk, yogurt, and cheese. There are also nondairy choices rich in calcium, such as sardines, tofu, and spinach.

MEAT, POULTRY, FISH, EGGS, BEANS, AND NUTS

These protein-rich foods form an important part of your diet and shouldn't be neglected in the quest to lower fat and cholesterol or reduce weight. Among the most important benefits these foods provide are amino acids to build and repair muscles, assure proper muscle development, and reduce the risk of iron-deficiency anemia.

The best low-fat, high-protein choices are: lean meat; fish, particularly salmon, tuna, swordfish, sardines, or bluefish; chicken or turkey with the skin removed; beans; legumes; and an increasingly popular option, protein-rich tofu. Prepare meat, poultry, and fish by broiling, baking, or grilling rather than frying.

A personal note:

Dinner is my main protein meal. Four times a week, I have chicken, meat, or fish. One night my dinner features eggs or cheese. The rest of the week I build dinner around pasta, although I often add some protein by using leftover chicken or meat.

FATS, OILS, AND SWEETS

There is a misperception that low-fat means no-fat. *That's not true and not good for you.* Fats, oils, and sweets sit on top of the nutrient pyramid because they should be used only in small amounts. But they are important to a balanced diet. They add taste, flavor, and a feeling of fullness, so you walk away from eating satisfied. Fats also help to transport fat-soluble vitamins such as A, D, E, and K and provide essential fatty acids the body can't produce itself.

What fats or sweets should you add to your diet? Among the best choices are olive oil for cooking and salad dressing, berry jams for sweetness, and walnuts. Also, it's okay to eat your favorite dessert occasionally. Many nutritionists now agree there are no totally "bad" foods, if they are used in moderation. So don't wage a losing battle with yourself about an occasional portion of ice cream, cake, or whatever you crave—just eat it in moderation as part of an overall balanced plan.

A personal note:

I don't believe in totally fat-free or even in very low-fat diets because I think that fat, carbohydrates, and proteins need to work together. Not only do you need fat for long-term energy, but if you cut out fat entirely or reduce it too much, you'll wind up feeling cold and very depressed. Balance is essential. If I crave a food I know is high in fat, I eat it. I've found it's better to satisfy that hunger when it hits me than to try to deny it. I don't ever feel the urge to binge!

How to Prepare Lower-Fat, Tasty Meals

The following menus are lower-fat and lower-calorie alternatives to traditional meals. These menus provide the balanced nutrients you need without adding empty calories, and they are tasty and satisfying. The ultimate goal is to eat food that is good for you without totally depriving yourself of food you enjoy.

MEAT MEAL

Traditional higher fat preparation	Lower fat preparation
Fried pork chops,	Grilled pork chops, fat trimmed
Pan gravy	Steamed potatoes, with skin, served with teaspoon of butter, chopped chives, and parsley
Mashed potatoes with butter	
Broccoli with hollandaise sauce	Steamed broccoli with sesame seeds
Ice cream with strawberries	Strawberries with vanilla yogurt and sugar or sugar substitute

PASTA MEAL

Traditional preparation

Spaghetti and sauce from a jar

Fried Italian sausages

Tossed salad with ranch dressing

Garlic bread

Italian Pastry

Lower fat preparation

Spaghetti and homemade sauce*

Tossed salad, lightly dressed with
olive oil and/or balsamic vinegar

Grilled bread lightly brushed with
olive oil and sprinkling of basil

Fresh fruit

OMELET BREAKFAST

Traditional preparation

Three egg omelet prepared with
milk and butter

Grated cheddar or gruyere cheese
in omelet

Honey buns or danish

Orange juice

Coffee

Lower fat preparation

Egg Beaters omelet prepared with
2 percent milk and canola oil or
nonstick spray

Grated mozzarella cheese and
chopped parsley filling for omelet

Whole wheat or rye toast and jam

Orange juice

---

*PREPARING YOUR OWN FAT-FREE PASTA SAUCE

Combine a large can of tomatoes, half a can of water, a handful of fresh, sweet basil or 1 tablespoon of dried basil, chopped onion, with any or all of the following: chopped mushrooms, eggplant, or spinach. Cook slowly for ten to fifteen minutes. You can add extra protein (and a slight amount of fat) to your pasta meal by adding sliced chicken, chopped tofu, or grated cheese when you serve the pasta.

Tips for Exercise-Friendly Eating

- **BEGIN THE DAY WITH A GOOD BREAKFAST.** Not only do breakfast foods provide essential nutrition, this meal starts your system off right. As I said, food is fuel, and after eight hours of sleep you need energy to get the day off to a good start. Once you eat, your metabolism revs up, as does your digestive system. You can eat a light breakfast—juice, fruit and plain, low-fat yogurt, a slice of toast or a bagel, and coffee or tea.

- **READ FOOD LABELS.** The "Nutrition Facts" food label required on all packaged foods helps you make good food choices. With such information as serving size, calories, fat content, protein, cholesterol, sodium, fiber, sugar, vitamins, and carbohydrates listed on the label, there is a wealth of information available.

    For instance, the "% Daily Values" shows how much a particular food, in a specific serving size, contributes to your overall daily requirements for the major nutrient areas. You can compare one food to another easily to create balanced meals that provide the nutrients you need without loading up on too much fat or sugar.

    Beware! Low-fat does not mean low-calorie. Always check the label for calories per portion of a food.

- **SET ASIDE TIME TO SHOP, SO YOU WON'T HAVE TO RESORT TO EMPTY CALORIES AND NUTRITION CHOICES IF YOU ARE RUNNING LATE.** Time management is as important to eating right as it is in finding time to exercise. Try to keep a stock of basic foods in the house and plan before you make trips to the supermarket or meat, fish, and produce vendors. By doing this, you'll be able to make up quick meals if you have to, and you'll have good ingredients to choose among.

Always stock up on the basics: pasta, spices, and canned foods. If you live in the suburbs or the country, sketch out a week's worth of meals, including breakfast and lunch, before you make your weekly trip to the supermarket. If you live in a city, where you have easier access to food vendors but less storage space, you may make two or three trips weekly to the markets. Try to avoid the ready-made takeout meal or restaurant food, as they are notoriously high in saturated fats. It helps if you have an eating plan in mind when the week begins.

- **IF YOU HAVE A CHOICE, BUY FRESH RATHER THAN PACKAGED FOODS.** When you place a premium on wholesome foods, it makes sense to start out with fresh ingredients. Packaged foods often have more fat, sugar, and sodium than you need. If you're pressed for time, prepared foods may be the best choice, but be selective. You can probably steam fresh vegetables in the time it takes to read the packaged food label. Be sure to read the label and maintain balance in your diet.

- **MAKE MORE THAN ONE MEAL TO SAVE TIME LATER.** This is a corollary to the previous point. When you're spending time in the kitchen to prepare meals for the next day or week, why not double up your preparations and freeze the extra? You'll make better use of your time and have food ready when you come home, so you won't be tempted to order takeout food or go to a restaurant instead.

- **BEWARE OF THE PITFALLS IN RESTAURANT EATING.** Although this point is often made when talking about weight-loss programs, it has a place here as well. Restaurant food almost always contains too much fat and too many calories. You can do the best job of controlling both these elements when you prepare food yourself.

    If you eat out, select your food carefully, ask how it is being prepared so you can make informed choices, and don't clean your plate since portions are usually *very* large. Take leftovers home with you—there's an easy lunch for the next day in almost all restaurant doggy bags.

Weight Control and Exercise

A personal note:

Diets alone don't work in losing weight and keeping it off because they stress the negative—what you can't or shouldn't do. To achieve something, you need to feel positive about your efforts, and that's what exercise provides— a powerful positive reinforcement that makes you happy with your body, not hate it.

Bring together any group of women over forty and you're likely to hear an abundance of "war stories" on efforts to lose weight. From liquid diets to pills, from carbohydrate counters to grapefruits and back again, the stories almost always end in failure and discouragement. Even professionals believe that those who have a lot of weight to lose and who have been overweight a long time are more likely than not to fail.

However, in *Thin for Life*, nutritionist Anne M. Fletcher recounted success stories of 160 patients, who managed to keep off at least 20 pounds for a minimum of three years. They didn't use a magic formula, drugs, or appetite suppressants. Nearly 90 percent of these patients lost weight by a combination of modified eating habits and increased exercise. Regular exercise alone won't do the trick, but it's a key part of the vast majority of success stories.

There are some basic truths about losing weight: Calories count, losing weight requires work, and you have to be patient—it won't happen overnight, no matter what fad diet proponents tell you. But there is one additional truth: The best way to achieve long-lasting weight loss is to combine new eating habits and exercise.

How does exercise promote weight loss? There are several ways:

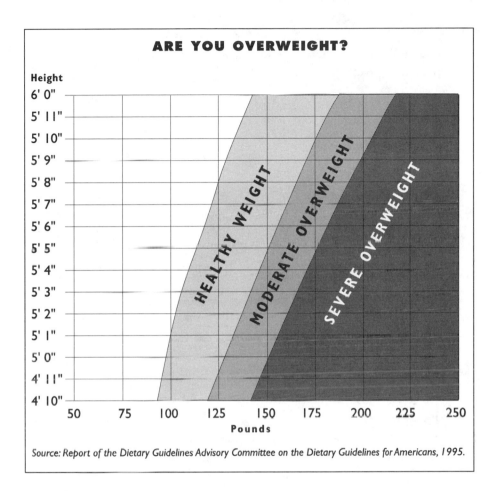

ARE YOU OVERWEIGHT?

Height

6' 0"
5' 11"
5' 10"
5' 9"
5' 8"
5' 7"
5' 6"
5' 5"
5' 4"
5' 3"
5' 2"
5' 1"
5' 0"
4' 11"
4' 10"

HEALTHY WEIGHT

MODERATE OVERWEIGHT

SEVERE OVERWEIGHT

50   75   100   125   150   175   200   225   250

Pounds

Source: Report of the Dietary Guidelines Advisory Committee on the Dietary Guidelines for Americans, 1995.

- Exercise burns fat.
- Exercise increases your rate of metabolism, which is the measure of how quickly your body uses up the calories needed to maintain daily activity.
- Exercise increases the size and tone of your muscles, and muscles use more calories than fat does.

Exercise also makes you feel better mentally. It relieves stress, gives you a sense of accomplishment, and fosters a better self-image—

all very helpful in keeping you motivated on a weight-loss program.

Once you see results from a combination of exercise and more healthful eating habits, you'll feel a natural reinforcement that will keep you on the right track. However, some people fall into a trap of overdoing things, either with eating or exercise.

Most doctors and nutritionists believe that a sensible weight-loss plan means that you lose about one pound a week and that you not be restricted to fewer than 1,200 calories a day. They also agree that you need to eat to lose weight, since the consumption of food raises the metabolic rate. Eating three proper meals a day, along with healthful snacks, will allow you to lose the weight you want to and keep it off.

Time after time, its been shown that *you can't starve yourself into being thin.* If you try the starvation method, your body simply slows down to protect itself; it's not getting enough calories to maintain itself. Any weight you lose will be slow going and quickly regained—and probably some more, since the body doesn't like being hungry.

In the same way, you shouldn't overdo your exercise program. If walking or running thirty minutes, plus doing some weight training, is allowing you to lose pounds, don't think that you'll get twice the results if you do twice the exercise. Doing too much exercise can lead to injury, fatigue, and irritability, and most likely your exercise program will screech to a halt. Even if you are running or walking primarily to help you lose weight, the activity itself should always be fun. If you want to increase time and distance or become competitive, do so gradually.

If you are committed to a weight-loss program, it makes sense to talk with a doctor or nutritionist before you begin. He or she can help you determine how many calories a day you should be eating in order to lose weight without feeling deprived and can help put together a sensible eating plan that includes a wide variety of food, full nutritional value, and tasty recipes.

You also don't need to try to go it alone. Besides the help those professionals can give you, there are commercial weight-loss programs such as Weight Watchers and Overeaters Anonymous, as well as university-based health and wellness programs, where you can join others who are learning to take control of their eating habits without relying on prepackaged meals or other gimmicks. Again, a training partner or group can be a great motivator in exercising.

A personal note:

I used to get a side stitch (cramp) only if I ate too soon before running. Interestingly, after forty, I started getting them also when running while I was totally famished. If I'm really hungry, I'll eat half a banana before I go out—I can run almost immediately after eating that.

Keeping Yourself Liquid: Water, Sports Drinks, Alcohol, and Caffeine

Water is one of the most easily overlooked parts of a healthful diet, particularly if you are active in sports. If you don't drink enough or lose too much liquid because of profuse sweating, it can affect your performance and leave you feeling less than your best.

We hardly take note of all the jobs water performs in our bodies: In the blood, water transports fats to muscles and carries away metabolic wastes such as carbon dioxide and lactic acid. In the urine, water eliminates waste. As sweat, water coats your skin and evaporates as you exercise, cooling the body. Throughout the body, water lubricates joints and cushions organs and tissues.

With all of that work to do, the body needs a constant resupply of liquid. Although feeling thirsty is usually a reliable gauge of how often to drink, it's not good enough when you're involved in regular workouts. Under these circumstances, we often don't drink sufficiently to replace the liquid lost during exercise. The best rule of thumb after exercise is to drink enough to quench your thirst and then a bit more.

Keeping yourself adequately hydrated involves three steps.

1. Drink enough every day. The typical recommendation of eight glasses of water a day is a good start, but when you're involved in regular aerobic exercise, you'll probably need up to an extra quart of water per day. The best way to keep track of whether you're drinking enough is to monitor your urine output. If you go to the bathroom every two or four hours and your urine is a light color, you're probably drinking enough.

2. Drink additional water before your workout. The amount depends on your size and how much your stomach can tolerate—usually a cupful is fine. You don't want to feel bloated when you start to walk or run.

3. Drink while you're exercising. If you're working out in hot weather, drink as much as you can as often as you can. Even in cooler weather, a tough workout makes you sweat, and you need to replace that fluid. Either carry fluids with you or, once your walk or run is over, start drinking to replace what you've lost.

Water is not your only fluid replacement choice. Juice, herbal tea, lemonade, sodium-free seltzer, skim milk, sports drinks, and low-sodium soup are also good additions. Colas and coffee or tea (hot or iced) are refreshing, but unless they are decaffeinated they cannot be considered fluid replacements. Caffeine is a diuretic that promotes fluid elimination, which you don't want. If you don't want to give up caffeine, be sure to add extra water to your fluid intake.

Still, coffee is a very popular drink among competitive runners. Most of them have a cup of coffee before a morning run to get their systems and bowels going. Before a race, most consider their cup of coffee essential.

Sports drinks have come into their own in recent years. They are designed to replace not only fluid but also the minerals and energy lost through sweating. Some sports drinks are reportedly absorbed more quickly than water, and rapidly replacing sweated-out minerals is an advantage. Read labels carefully because some of these magical performance-enhancing elixirs are high in calories and may not be worthwhile for moderate-level exercisers who are also looking to lose weight. They replace energy and the taste may be better than water in some areas.

On the horizon are performance-enhancing versions of sports drinks made with a combination of minerals and carbohydrates. If they help you stay fluid, drink them!

For many runners, the postrace beer is considered a part of the sport's ritual. While alcohol in moderation won't adversely affect your performance, it's best to save beer and wine for meals and relaxation time. Alcohol dehydrates (and disorients!) you, so it's not advised at all before exercising. After a workout, be sure to drink water before and then along with your beer or wine to get the fluid replacement you require.

chapter 10

YOUR CHANGING BODY

MENOPAUSE, EXERCISE, AND AGING HAPPILY

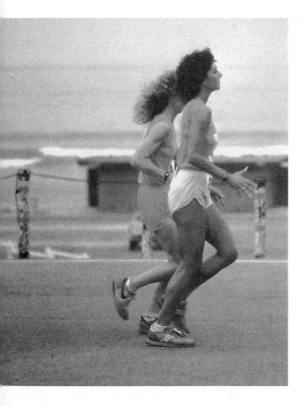

A personal note:

All my life I've been an athlete, or had an athlete's mentality about keeping fit. Keeping a balance between my body and my mind was critical to my sense of self. As long as I trained, my body would respond to the goals I set. I never thought that would change. However, when I reached menopause, I discovered that my body had its own agenda. At first I felt betrayed. Once I understood what was happening, I did something about it. I continue to be fit and athletic. These were—and still are—the most important things I can do to keep my body and mind in balance and my sense of self intact. And you can do them too!

One thing's certain: The longer you live, the older you get. We joke about aging, feel depressed about it, and valiantly try to forestall the process. Very few of us delight in it. Yet getting older can bring some of the best years of our lives offering possibility, freedom, and insight we never had before.

Too many women feel that aging ends their attractiveness, usefulness, and capability. They fall victim to the myth that our youth-obsessed world and culture has passed them by. Bombarded by media images of sexy young models airbrushed to perfection, competition seems hopeless.

Since the average woman today can expect to live a third of her life after age forty, she needs to realize that there are benefits to aging. Shedding the pressures and expectations of youth allows you to be yourself, explore new territory (physical or mental), and unlock creativity. This sense of freedom can make you soar.

The secret to making your later years your happiest rests in two words: health and attitude.

You don't have to stand by watching your health profile change beyond your control or recognition. Regular exercise helps you maintain your figure. It also lowers the risk of many cancers, diabetes, high blood pressure, and heart attack. Weight bearing exercises such as running and walking build and maintain bone, a key element in reducing the risk or severity of osteoporosis. And it's been medically proven that bones and muscles respond positively to exercise at *any* age.

Embrace change in a positive manner instead of fighting it. You don't have to be a victim. You can do more to help yourself than you may realize. Again, exercise—running and walking in particular—plays a crucial role. Sustained aerobic exercise (the kind that makes you breathe deeply and sweat) releases natural chemical mood enhancers called endorphins into the system, making you feel good and giving you a sense of optimism. It breaks the cycle of depression that often comes with aging by helping you to build a positive outlook about yourself and the future.

Valuable help is also available from the medical profession, organizations devoted to women's health issues, books, magazines, and friends.

If you're troubled by the changes in your body, start doing something about it now. Fitness gives you a positive hold on both health and attitude.

A personal note:

You'll never see a happier group of people than the ones I find in over-forty (or fifty, sixty, seventy, or even eighty) fitness groups. At my first World Veterans Track and Field Championships, I was stunned by the quality of the performances and the attitude of the athletes. None of the men or women wished he or she was twenty-five again. They were living totally in the present. Unconcerned about being younger, they enjoyed tough competition in their age groups and even had the energy to party like mad when the competition was over.

Changes: What and Why

Aging alters the life you have been living in subtle and profound ways. Kids grow up and leave home, job retirement is on the horizon, illness or death may come to a spouse, partner, or friend, and you begin to experience physical and emotional changes. All of these work together in changing how you live.

Most of us find the physical changes particularly unsettling. For years we take our bodies for granted. Perhaps there are few more lines and wrinkles that cause you to joke about giving yourself a face-lift at fifty. Or you may feel less resilient and unable to do all the things you could just a few years before. But we rarely give serious thought to how our bodies have already been changing, even in our forties.

Then, in what feels like an instant, the wheels fall off and nothing about your body functions in the same way. We're always surprised. Most of these physical changes occur because of one big event:

Menopause. Shrouded for so long in mystery and myth, it not surprising many women don't want to say the word and just refer to it as the change.

The Change

Menopause means your period stops, right? That's what I thought: Periods end, another inconvenience is behind me. Wouldn't it be great if it were so easy?

Even though menopause is a natural process, it is not a simple one. Cessation of the menstrual period is just one of many complex things happening to your body before, during, and after menopause. Many women bear the changes with hardly a ripple, but for millions of others, the physical and emotional transformations of menopause are devastating Although I believe menopause should be embraced with happiness, and even honor, those are probably the *last* things many of us feel.

While the end of menstruation is the classic sign of menopause, it is also the time when your ovaries stop releasing eggs, and there is a sharp decline in the production of estrogen and other ovarian hormones. It is the end of fertility. For some women these occur all at once; for other they happen gradually.

Perimenopause is the name for the transitional cycle leading to menopause that women begin to experience three to five years before their periods end. A variety of physical symptoms associated with menopause actually begin during perimenopause because of declining levels of reproductive hormones. These can include hot flashes and profuse sweating, intense feelings of heat followed by intense feelings of cold, and vaginal dryness.

The decline in production of estrogen during perimenopause can cause emotional ups and down that are very much like those experienced during adolescence. But many of us find these feelings more intense at this stage of life because they are bound up in conflicting feelings about aging, the loss of reproductive function, and the many other midlife changes that are taking place at this time.

As a result, it is often difficult to tell if your moods and physical state are due to chemical changes or happenstance. Are you feeling sad and useless because your children are leaving home or because hormonal changes are making you depressed? Are you feeling less sexy and attractive because you know intellectually you cannot reproduce or because chemical changes have altered your libido? Are you always tired because physical changes are affecting your sleep or because you're in a plateau with your job? Chances are these feelings are due to a combination of these factors and the reasons can't be easily delineated.

A personal note:

I'm really saddened when I see menopausal women who, when depressed, turn to alcohol or tranquilizers. It could be simply that they are lacking estrogen. I further believe that a lot of memory loss occurs for this reason, and there are exciting new studies showing that dementia and even Alzheimer's may be reduced with hormone replacement therapy. A daily run sure helps! Plenty of depressed people experience an emotional lift from exercising.

What Happens During Menopause

Mother Nature didn't intend for most animals, including us, to outlive their reproductive usefulness. Because of advances in medical science, this is the first century in history where the life expectancy of women is over age fifty. Not content merely to live past menopause, ours is the first generation of women who expect to continue to live healthily, active, even sexy lives after reproductive function is over. We are truly rewriting history!

Here are the basics: Women are born with ovaries filled with thousands of eggs. (Nature usually overcompensates; she wants to make *sure* that you can reproduce!) At puberty, the pituitary gland in the brain begins releasing follicle-stimulating hormone (FSH), causing the ovaries to release an egg every month. At the same time, the uterus builds up a lining of blood and nutrient tissue in anticipation of the egg being fertilized (pregnancy). Most of the eggs are not fertilized and are shed each month, along with the lining of the uterus, as menstrual blood.

As we age, our eggs age too and then die off. This occurs around age fifty. Stress, pollution, poor nutrition, and other factors may also contribute to the eggs diminishing and dying earlier. During perimenopause, our brain works harder, releasing more FSH to get the ovaries to continue to release eggs. The lining of the uterus may build up greater than ever, and menstrual flow is often extremely, and distressingly, heavy. Some periods are skipped altogether. Premenstrual syndrome (PMS), irritability, and moodiness can worsen or appear when you have never experienced it before. The hypothalamus gland of the brain, which regulates temperature, is also affected, sometimes causing uncontrollable rises in temperature and sweating known as hot flashes or hot flushes.

Eventually, the brain gives up when there are no more eggs, and the uterus also ceases its monthly buildup of its lining. Thus, there are no more menstrual periods, and at this point, the ovaries begin to cease producing the hormone estrogen. This is menopause, and this seems to be where real distress occurs: The lack of estrogen causes a chemical shift in the body, and for many the symptoms are very similar to drug withdrawal: headaches, night sweats, bad dreams, broken sleep or insomnia, chronic fatigue, depression, gastrointestinal upset, and, perhaps most frightening of all, memory loss. It's no wonder that many menopausal women (and their partners) think they are losing their minds. And it's confusing because these are all also symptoms of extreme stress, which may be occurring anyway because of the other midlife changes we've discussed.

Coping with Menopause

Fortunately, most of us can weather these changes with equanimity, but for others they seem overwhelming. One place to turn for help is your gynecologist. Although some women believe that doctors incorrectly characterize menopause as a disease to be treated rather than as a natural part of the aging process, many women need specific relief that's available now only from their doctors. There is also a great deal of evidence that medical intervention—along with your own health and fitness program—can help prevent many problems and risks associated with aging. My personal experience is that a daily walk or run can be physically and emotionally lifesaving, and this is a simple, easy, and even discreet decision that puts *you* back in control of your body. Like menopause itself, the solutions that work for you may be varied and complex.

Osteoporosis and Heart Disease: More Transitions

OSTEOPOROSIS

Although most of the common symptoms of menopause eventually can be overcome by braving them out or using medication, the danger of osteoporosis and heart disease is quite different. Osteoporosis is often called the silent disease because there are no specific symptoms to treat. It occurs when there is a severe loss of bone density, thinning of bone tissue, and the growth of small holes in the bone. The combination of these changes results in bones that are thinner, more porous, and more breakable.

The link between osteoporosis and menopause is the fact that the cessation of estrogen production can cause severe loss in bone density in a short period of time. Women can lose up to 20 percent of their bone mass in the five to seven years after menopause, making us more susceptible to osteoporosis. The risk is highest for thin white women who smoke and/or drink excessively and who have a family history of osteoporosis, and for women who enter menopause early. At the present time, one postmenopausal woman in three is developing or already has severe bone loss, a $10 billion-a-year problem that results in 1.3 million fractures and thousands of deaths each year.

Bones strengthen at any age with use, but the sooner you begin to exercise the better it is for your future. But exercise alone may not be enough to forestall osteoporosis. Lack of estrogen is devastating on bones, and studies have established that use of estrogen early in menopause can cut the risk of fractures in half.

To find out your risk for osteoporosis, include a baseline bone scan to measure bone density in your regular checkup. Estrogen replacement therapy and increasing calcium intake are two of the most effective ways to forestall further bone loss. Weight-bearing exercise, such as walking, running, and strength training, is also important to keep bones strong. In addition, exercise improves coordination and helps prevent the falls that are so dangerous to women suffering from the disease.

HEART DISEASE

Women seem virtually immune to heart attacks when they are young. Heart disease is mostly a man's problem until women become menopausal. Then, postmenopausal women have the same rates of heart disease as men. Estrogen seems to protect women from heart disease, but when estrogen stops, cholesterol levels rise, the arteries become narrow and less elastic, and blood clots form more easily.

Running and walking are ideal in this situation because they not only increase cardiovascular capacity but also help expand major arteries. In addition, taking estrogen replacement may be a big benefit in preventing future heart disease. A 1995 study in the *New England Journal of Medicine* revealed that women who continue hormone replacement therapy (HRT) for five or more years after menopause reduce their risk of developing heart disease by 50 percent. That's pretty dramatic and for many women overrides the risks associated with HRT.

Dealing with Menopause and Medical Options

Today women can reverse some of the unwelcome side effects of menopause by taking hormonal supplements to replace the estrogen their bodies no longer produce. These hormones can be administered orally or by a time-release adhesive patch. But these options are not without some serious drawbacks. Physicians have debated the pros and cons of estrogen supplements for decades; at present, the majority are clearly on the side of taking them, at least for most women.

Like genetic engineering and other advancements in medicine, hormone replacement therapy is an attempt to improve on nature's design. When it first became popular several decades ago, women were given rather large doses of estrogen daily, a one-size-fits-all approach later found to result in a ninefold increase in the risk of uterine cancer. To protect the uterus against cancer, the regimen was changed to cyclical hormone therapy, which meant lower doses of estrogen for twenty-five days of the month, then the synthetic hormone progestin (progesterone) for the last ten of those twenty-five days, and nothing for the last five days.

Cyclical hormone therapy more closely mimics a woman's natural cycle, which means that menstrual bleeding often continues for years beyond menopause. In addition, when progestin is given, some women have enough side effects—such as bloating, depression, and irritability—to convince them to abandon hormone treatment.

Then there's the possibility of an increased risk of breast cancer, which physicians and researchers are still trying to assess. The studies conducted have offered no conclusive results. Some have shown no increased risk associated with hormone replacement and others a rise of about 35 percent in the risk.

While we know that estrogen alone can increase the risk of endometrial cancer, combining estrogen and progesterone appears to eliminate this risk. What's not certain is whether adding progestin also protects the breasts against cancer or diminishes the benefits of estrogen to the heart.

We do know that *heart disease kills four times more women than breast cancer does.* In women younger than seventy-five, there are more than three times as many deaths from heart disease than from breast cancer. So even if the hormone therapy somewhat increases risk of breast cancer, it still represents a substantial overall benefit. But that judgment may differ for women at particular risk of this cancer.

Advances in Hormone Replacement Therapy

There are now many choices available in hormone therapy: different dosages, different hormone combinations, and different methods of administering them. This means that replacement therapy can be better tailored to individual needs. Especially promising are the compounds known as SERMs (selective estrogen-receptor modulators), so-called "designer estrogen."

Estrogen initially was viewed as something that would affect a woman's bones, breasts, heart, and uterus as if a single molecular switch was being turned on all over the body whenever the hormone was taken. But scientists testing the drug tamoxifen on women with breast cancer discovered something unexpected. Because tamoxifen was supposed to turn off the estrogen switch, a woman with breast cancer would take it on the theory that starving breast tissue of natural estrogen would help shrink or prevent tumors. It was assumed that if there was no estrogen going to the breasts there would be none going to the bones either, meaning that the bone quality in women on tamoxifen would not be good. In fact, the women's bones were fine. Tamoxifen was turning off the estrogen switch in the breasts but was still acting just like estrogen in the bones, suggesting the possibility that estrogen didn't work the same way in every cell. This, in turn, gave rise to potentially being able to build compounds that would be tissue selective.

Researchers currently believe there are many estrogen switches in the body and that turning them on or off depends on the type of the estrogenlike compound that is taken. There is a second generation of

SERMs now in development that act like estrogen in the heart and the bones but block the harmful effects of estrogen in the breasts and the uterus. In the conceivable future, women worried about raising their breast cancer risk may have the option of taking a different kind of hormone that doesn't affect their breasts, or that may protect against breast cancer.

Finally, at the end of 1997, the Food and Drug Administration approved a synthetic estrogen that seems to offer the benefits of estrogen without increasing the risks of cancer.

In short, women have always had to make their decision based on a comparison of risks and benefits, but now the risks and benefits are changing because more selective estrogen compounds are coming along that will offer alternatives.

A personal note:

> *Many women lash out at the medical community for not treating menopause with natural remedies such as Chinese herbs as if doctors are some kind of patriarchy dictating the terms of our bodies to us. I believe that part of a positive attitude about menopause allows us to take knowledge from a variety of sources.*

Hormone replacement therapy now seems effective and fairly safe. With no hormone replacement therapy, the typical American woman faces more than a third of her life without the benefits of estrogen to her heart, bones, skin, and other tissues.

Other Views, Other Choices

Despite this, the majority of menopausal women do not choose to take replacement hormones. For many, the inducement of benefits to heart and bones is not worth continuing to take replacement hormones for the seven or more years needed. Once women have passed through menopause and the more disturbing menopausal symptoms cease, they discontinue taking these hormones.

Some women question the wisdom of tampering with the body's chemistry and are against treating a natural passage in life as a "medical problem." Others fear that hormone replacement therapy will increase their risk of developing breast or uterine cancer, or will promote the growth of a preexisting cancer.

What about women who do not choose to take hormone replacements or, for one reason or another, cannot? Are exercise and diet alone enough to offset any damage menopause may precipitate?

There are physicians, practitioners of alternative medicine, and authors of health books who believe that exercise and a good diet are all that matter, that medicine cannot help us if we do not first help ourselves. This line of thought may inspire people to take themselves in hand, which is all to the good.

Women should, without question, exercise, eat properly, and take charge of their lives. We should all learn to listen to our bodies and make our own choices. But there are going to be times when that won't be sufficient, when what we learn and what we accomplish don't begin to compare to what we don't know and can't do. That's the time to consult physicians and allow medicine to help.

Of course, it would be easier to make choices if all the facts about the various options were available. Not even the now-standard cyclical therapy has been adequately tested for long-term benefits to the heart, blood vessels, and bones and for long-term complications.

Properly designed studies are under way, but the results will not be available for about ten years, by which time millions more women will have entered menopause and grappled with a decision about whether and how to treat it. In the absence of definitive answers, most experts agree that the best approach is for each woman and her doctor to review her risk factors and family medical history, talk about her concerns, and the therapeutic options available. Then, together come to an informed decision.

Whatever your choice regarding hormone-replacement therapy,

there is every good reason to tailor a fitness and nutrition program for yourself. Even if diet and exercise alone cannot *replicate* the benefits of estrogen replacement therapy, they can *enhance* it.

Lastly, many women gain weight taking estrogen. An informal survey among my friends estimates five to ten pounds, which is not a terrible price for feeling better, but it is annoying for those of us who try to keep fit. Maintaining an exercise program of walking and running substantially reduces any weight gain.

A personal note:

I weighed the risks of breast cancer against the benefits in preventing heart disease and osteoporosis, and, mathematically, HRT was quite an overwhelming winner. But the real reason I began on HRT was the need to regain control over my life: I felt depressed, forgetful, and indecisive. My hot flashes were unbearable and my skin crawled. The only time I felt normal was when I ran, but even I can't run twenty-four hours a day! HRT is not perfect. I hate taking drugs. I hate the weight gain that accompanies them, even though my running keeps that under control. Justified or not, I still blame HRT for every headache I get. But every day we learn more, and soon we'll get it right. In the meantime, my daily run still continues to be the day's salvation, the time when no matter what else, I feel like I always did . . . maybe just a little slower!

Tips for Dealing with Hot Flashes, Night Sweats, and Other Signs of Aging

- **HOT FLASHES AND NIGHT SWEATS.** Wear clothes in layers to peel off quickly. Keep a fan nearby. Drink hot liquids slowly, or replace them with iced drinks. Reduce your intake of alcohol. End each shower with a cool rinse. Keep natural fibers against the skin—this includes all-cotton sheets. Keep a window open for cool fresh air at night. Have a couple of very thin blankets on the bed rather than one heavy one. Make blankets easy to kick off your feet.

- **FACIAL HAIR AND ACNE.** With a lack of estrogen to inhibit it, the male hormone testosterone comes on strong, encouraging sprouting facial hairs (just where you don't want hair!) and often acne. HRT can reverse this; barring that, waxing, plucking, and topical acne treatment medications are best.

- **DRY, THINNING HAIR.** Just where you *do* want hair, the same testosterone works in reverse on the top of your head. Massage your scalp with oil and treat hair carefully.

- **DRY SKIN AND SCALY LEGS.** Use lots of lotion. If you are pale, add one of the new self-tanning creams to legs for a healthy appearance. Massage your body with lotion to get circulation going and bring blood to skin surface. Don't stay in a hot shower or bath too long. Put a humidifier device on your furnace, or put a humidifier in each room.

- **WRINKLES.** Stay out of the sun, always use a sunblock, and moisturize several times a day with a quality product.

- **SAGGING MUSCLES AND STIFF JOINTS.** In addition to the programs and exercises described here, you could try regular massage therapy or take up yoga at your local community center, yoga center, or gym.

- **VARICOSE VEINS.** Wear support hose and keep feet elevated as much as possible. Discuss options for vein removal or shrinkage with your doctor. Exercise is important to keep blood circulating. Severe varicose veins are more than an appearance problem; they are a health hazard, as they can often form blood clots.

- **COLD HANDS AND FEET.** Wear pure wool or cotton socks and gloves and keep moving. Running or walking is the perfect way to keep in motion and increase circulation.

- **GAS AND BLOATING.** Eat smaller meals more frequently. Keep moving; don't sit in one place for a long time. I recommend following your evening meal with a dose of Metamucil or taking Bean-O with gas-producing food.

- **GUT CRAMP.** Replace tight belts and waistbands with soft elastic; avoid constrictive panty hose and girdles. Avoid getting famished and then eating rapidly, especially while wearing tight panty hose. Again, I recommend Metamucil to keep gut expanded to avoid kinks and cramping. Keep regular with exercise, lots of water, and bran products. Wait an hour to run or walk after eating.

- **HEAVY MENSTRUAL FLOW.** Wear a tampon, heavy pad, and black tights. Since the worst flow usually occurs on day one of your period, you may want to make this your day off from running or walking.

- **HEARING LOSS.** Avoid loud places, wear ear plugs on airplanes, and try to avoid restaurants and other public spaces with loud background noise.

- **DIMINISHED VISION/IRRITATED EYES.** Get your eyes checked regularly eye checks, particularly for glaucoma. Use artificial tears and lubricants. Wear sunglasses in bright light. Use adequate lighting when reading or working at the computer. Get someone else to drive at night or call a taxi.

- **STRESS INCONTINENCE.** The muscles in your pelvic area may start to weaken. Do crunch sit-ups, practice sucking your abdomen in and holding it for a count of five several times a day, and especially start doing Kegel exercises (below), which are designed to strengthen vaginal walls.

  - Contract the vagina as if you are stopping a flow of urine.
  - Tighten the muscles a little and count to five.

- Tighten them a bit more and count to five.
- Tighten them as much as you can and count to five.
- Slowly release. Repeat five times.

Do Kegels several times a day.

Drink cranberry juice, try to urinate before exercise, wear dark tights or shorts.

- **DIMINISHED BLADDER CAPACITY.** Do your Kegels and drink most of your fluid during the day so you can sleep through the night.

- **DIMINISHED LIBIDO.** Feel good about yourself, exercise to raise endorphins and to strengthen and maintain your own body image, spend more time with your partner doing fun things, read erotic literature, paint the bedroom pink, and turn down the lights. If this doesn't work, talk to your doctor about possible drug treatment.

- **PAINFUL SEX/DRY VAGINA.** Lubricants help a lot—like Replens or Astroglide—but frequent sex is the best remedy to keep a thinning and shortening vagina flexible and lubricated. If all else fails, HRT may also help.

Final Thoughts About Change

Eventually, we'll come out the other end of menopause happy and wise. Maybe we'll even discover the "postmenopausal zest" that we keep hearing about. We're living beings; therefore we're always changing. It's important to realize that exercise and activity can not only help you through these changes but also can be the start of the whole new life that this era opens.

chapter 11

SAFETY WHILE RUNNING AND WALKING

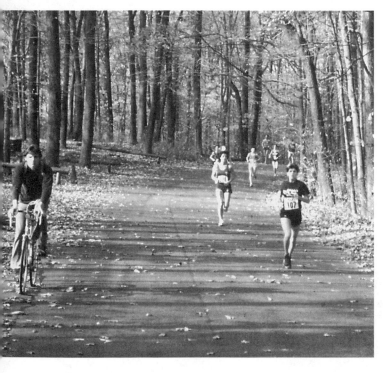

It's a sad but true fact of life that we have to be aware of our own safety when we run and walk. Unfortunately, attacks on women runners and walkers are on the increase largely because there are more women running and walking.

Actually, when you consider the thousands and thousands of women who run and walk every day in such supposedly "dangerous" places as Central Park, the assault statistics are so low as to be remarkable. Nevertheless, it always pays to be safe.

Body Language: A Powerful Tool for Self-Protection

When we're walking home from work or walking to our car in a dark or deserted parking lot, we're totally aware of the dangers that surround us. But when we're out exercising, we feel indestructible. This is one of the joys of exercise—it frees us. Sadly, when we are lost in thought and feeling free, what we often signal to predators is someone who is vulnerable and easily surprised. However, we can say just the opposite—that we are connected and powerful. What you convey through body language when you run can be as important as the neighborhood that you choose to run in or the risks that you decide to take.

It may sound like an empty slogan to tell women, "Hey! when you run or walk, do it POWERFULLY!" But the following true story shows how the mind can control body language in an important way. A policewoman was dressed to look like an elderly lady for decoy duty to attract muggers. She was a failure for a long time. Films revealed that nobody mugged her because she just looked like who she was: a very strong woman, too strong to attack.

What that means for you is that when you look strong, you *are* strong. Run or walk with your head up, shoulders back, eyes focused around you, and arms and legs swinging purposefully and striding strong. In short, good running and walking form sends a powerful message to would-be attackers that you're in control. Watch yourself run or walk in a storefront window to get an idea of how you look when you run and the message your body language is sending.

Although you should be careful throughout your run, take extra care at the beginning of a workout, when you're moving slowly and warming up. Perhaps you are literally just waking up or coming from a hectic day at home or in the office and are preoccupied; these are difficult times to concentrate on anything! The next most vulnerable time during your workout—both for potential assaults and injury—is at the end, when you are tired. Your mind starts to wander and you start to show fatigue. You can misjudge steps, curbs, and traffic. At times like this, it's good to say out loud to yourself, "Pay attention! Pay attention!"

DO'S AND DON'TS OF SAFE RUNNING AND WALKING

Henley Gabeau, the executive director of the Road Runners Club of America (RRCA), has been waging a safety campaign for women runners and walkers. Here are some of Henley's basic cautions, as well as a few others that have been shown to work for women runners and walkers.

- Always stay alert. The more aware you are, the less vulnerable you are.

- Don't wear headphones! Use your ears to be aware of your surroundings.

- Write down or leave word with someone of the direction of your walk or run.

- Tell friends and family about your favorite routes.

- Run or walk in familiar areas. In unfamiliar areas, contact a local RRCA chapter or running or walking store. Know where telephones are along the route or where there are open businesses or stores.

- Avoid unpopulated areas, deserted streets, and overgrown trails. Especially avoid unlit areas at night. Run clear of parked cars or bushes.

- Carry identification or write your name, phone number, blood type, and an emergency contact with telephone number on a tag you tie on your shoes. Also include important medical information.

- Don't wear jewelry.

- **Ignore verbal harassment. Use discretion in acknowledging strangers. Look directly at others and be observant but keep your distance and keep moving.**

- **Use your intuition about a person or an area. React on your intuitions and avoid someone or someplace if you're unsure.**

- **Practice memorizing license tags or identifying characteristics of strangers.**

- **Carry a whistle or other noisemaker.**

- **Call police immediately if something happens to you or someone else, or you notice anything out of the ordinary.**

General Safety Tips

Don't be afraid to be afraid. If something looks suspicious, turn and go in another direction. Too many of us think that we'll look like wimps; in fact, nobody cares.

Don't persist in running in a place that always makes you uncomfortable and wary. Beautiful but isolated trails lose their beauty if you're too nervous to enjoy them. Plus you'll find yourself becoming tense, not relaxed, defeating part of the purpose for running.

Check out any wooded area for wildlife that could be dangerous. Most of us know animals only in a zoo; in the wild they are not pets. Mountain lions are making a strong comeback in Colorado, grizzlies have been known to attack in our national parks, and an alligator can outrun a human. Watch your footing in snake country. These attacks are rare, but they can happen.

It's more likely you will encounter a barking dog than any other animal. Dogs may be woman's best friend, but they are often not a runner or walker's. Usually a dog is only protecting its territory; give it a wide berth and it generally won't attack. Most dogs are full of scary bluster—that's their job. But if a dog is aggressive, face it, meet its eyes, and stand still "like a tree" until it loses interest and goes away or back slowly away from it. Do not turn and run, as the dog's instinct is to give chase and bite. Be very careful with German shepherds and Dobermans, which are commonly trained as watchdogs. As for rottweilers and pit bulls, say some prayers too. If you know of neighborhoods where these breeds are unleashed, call the police immediately. If dogs really are a problem to you, and you cannot change your route or leash laws do not apply, try calling the owners. Tell them when you are going out and ask if they would tie up their dog for the next hour. Failing that, carry a can of dog mace.

Keep a pair of old running or walking shoes in the back of your car, with socks, a white shirt, and walking pants. Cars have a habit of breaking down at midnight in bad neighborhoods when you are in a cocktail dress. When you can't call for help, sometimes you can run or walk for it.

Even if you live alone, leave a note in an obvious place saying where you have gone walking or running, when you left, and when you expect to get back.

Don't become too predictable about when you run or walk. Occasionally, vary your route and the time of day you go out to exercise.

If a driver asks for directions, keep a safe distance from the car when you talk to him or her. Don't ever get in a car. Turn and run or walk away and look for other runners or walkers or somewhere to get help.

Running or Walking at Night

- Wear reflective clothing and a white shirt.
- Walk only where there is a sidewalk or really big shoulder of the road. Walk facing traffic and give it plenty of berth.
- Wear a white baseball hat so that the car headlights don't blind you.
- Make sure you know your route very well. If you can't see cracks in the sidewalk or holes in the road, you'll trip.

- It's best to walk with a partner or a leashed dog when you exercise at night. If you absolutely cannot, then put your hair up in a cap and look as much like a man as possible.

- Stick close to home. While nothing is perfectly safe, it is much safer running around your suburban or city block in the dark, where you know all your neighbors, than running a few miles away from home and then running back.

- Consider finding an indoor track, using a treadmill, or doing aerobics that night.

- A course in self-defense is helpful. You'll learn how to recognize and avoid danger and way to escape from bad situations. But don't be fooled into believing you can overpower a man. You can't do it. Period.

- If you are attacked, scream your head off and kick your legs to try to scare off your attacker. Even though you may not be able to overpower him, attackers may run away if you create a disturbance.

- I've said it before, but it's worth repeating: DON'T WEAR HEADPHONES when exercising outdoors. A huge proportion of women who are assaulted while running or walking were wearing headphones. You cannot hear someone coming up behind you, or cars or sirens. Worst of all, you cannot hear the birds, the wind, or your own heart beating!

A personal note:

Once, I was running along the bike trail near my home in Virginia there was a young woman in front of me running, wearing headphones. I decided to try something: I began running very closely behind her, only one step away. I ran for a mile like that, almost stepping on her heels, and I even flicked her ponytail a few times, just to see how alert she was. No reaction! When we got to an intersection, we stopped, and she was startled to see that I was right alongside of her. I'm mad at myself for not reading her the riot act because my words might save her life someday.

chapter 12

DON'T LET INJURIES SPOIL YOUR FUN

HOW TO PREVENT THEM AND WHAT TO DO IF THEY HAPPEN

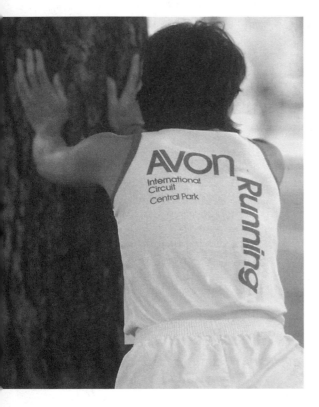

A personal note:

Whenever I've gotten hurt it's because I pushed myself and did something stupid that I should have known better than to attempt. The irony is that if we are going to get better—go faster and farther—in our running or walking, we need to push beyond our comfort zones. And that's where injury can lurk. However, if we are all sensible about equipment and training, we should enjoy many fabulous, injury-free miles running and walking.

Once you decide to start a running or walking program, you just want to get out there and do it—an understandable feeling that we all share. The running and walking programs outlined in

Chapters 3 and 4 provide a model to follow to achieve your fitness goals in a safe and healthful manner.

Enthusiasm is a wonderful thing. But as in so many other areas of life, when you approach your fitness program, you need to temper that excitement with sensible precautions. Although some *traumatic* injuries occur as a result of running or walking, the vast majority of injuries associated with these activities are what the medical profession calls *overuse* injuries. What's the difference? A turned ankle, a fall, a twist to your leg from stepping in a hole, or overstretching a low back muscle are all traumatic injuries. They occur suddenly and, depending on their severity, may need immediate medical treatment or rest.

Overuse injuries such as tendonitis or stress fractures can occur several ways. If you train beyond your level of fitness, do too much too soon, wear faulty shoes, or ignore warning signals your body is giving you, you may be vulnerable to this type of injury. Overuse injuries are far more likely than traumatic injuries, and they almost always develop slowly and are often preventable if we are careful in our training methods and become aware of changes in our body or the persistance of little hurts that we often exercise through. These may be warning signs of a developing injury and shouldn't be ignored.

Guidelines for Preventing Injuries

CHOOSE THE RIGHT SHOES, YOUR FIRST LINE OF PROTECTION AGAINST INJURY

A lot of injuries occur because you don't have the proper shoes or your shoes are worn out. If they are not the right shoe for your foot type or for the kind of exercise you are doing, you may be exposing yourself to preventable problems. How to determine your foot type and the shoe choices available to fit you properly are outlined in Chapter 5 on equipment. Once you've decided on the type of shoe you need, don't be shy about trying on a variety of brands, testing the shoes, and asking the salesperson lots of questions about fit and shoe features. It's your most important fitness purchase, so take your time buying shoes. The payoff is enormous.

After you've started to run or walk regularly, routinely examine your shoes for wear. Be prepared to replace your shoes after about four hundred to five hundred miles of use or at least every year, if you run or walk three times a week. Also, look for wear patterns on the soles. A thorough check of the inside of the shoe is important, as well.

A personal note:

Shoes can begin to bottom out and feel flat from the normal pressing down that comes with running and walking on all surfaces. There is a really profound loss of shock absorption. I don't know how many times I've heard runners working out in new shoes say, "Oh, I feel like I'm floating on air," and suddenly they realize they have been running in worn-down shoes, even when they look fine from the outside.

BEGIN GRADUALLY

This is an important area to keep in mind both for your daily workouts and your overall program. When you start a workout, do it slowly. If you are running, begin by walking and then gradually move into easy jogging for a few minutes while you try to get the kinks out or shrug off some stiffness. Walkers should also begin at an easy tempo and steadily build up to their training pace. A rough indicator of when you're warmed up is when you start to sweat.

Slow and steady at the beginning is also a good approach to your overall exercise program. Dr. Joe Miller, a professor of orthopedics at New York Chiropractic College in Seneca Falls, New York, encourages many of his patients to start walking programs but cautions them to be realistic about how quickly they will see changes. "I want my patients to think long-term," Dr. Miller says. "It takes some eight to ten weeks to see results from a walking program. And there is no benefit to trying to speed up the process. That's how you expose yourself to the possibility of injury."

If weight loss is a major goal of your running or walking program, Dr. Ayne Furman says patience is vital. "Changes will come, but it might take as much as three months before you will see them. It is important to understand this and not give up too soon."

LISTEN TO YOUR BODY

Listening to your body is not an idea pulled from a New Age philosophy or the suggestion that running or walking will take you to a higher level of consciousness. It means you need to be aware of how your body feels during exercise. Learn to trust your instincts and intuition. Your body will give you signals about how it feels with the work you are doing. It will also let you know if it is happy or unhappy with the stress you are placing on it. Look for these signs, which often come in the form of discomfort, pain, or fatigue, and pay attention to them.

Once you are aware of a change in how you feel, you need to determine why it's happened. Have you injured yourself? Or are you more tired and sore than normal because of extra exertion you are placing on your body in an effort to improve your performance? Anytime you push yourself you are going to experience some slight discomfort. You may be more tired after your workout and the next day or two you might feel new soreness in your muscles. You need to be running for only about a month to be able to tell right away the difference between an injury and the sense of discomfort caused by extra effort.

A personal note:

I love the pleasant sense of fatigue that comes after a hard workout. The next day my muscles twinge, then two days later they feel a bit sore. I take it easy those days and am ready again on day three. This sense of fatigue makes me feel as if I have accomplished something—that I'm going farther and making progress in my training. It's a very different feeling from the hurt of an oncom-

ing injury. When I feel like that, I stop immediately and check out the reason. You'll soon know the difference between these two sensations.

An unusual or severe pain will automatically cause you to stop what you are doing, but other signals may be more subtle and difficult to read. Here are some warning signs you should be aware of. They show that something is happening that requires your attention before continuing your running or walking.

WARNING SIGNALS

- **Mild tenderness, muscle stiffness, or limping that does not go away after a few days of rest**
- **Muscle cramping or spasm during or after exercise**
- **Swelling or redness in any area**
- **Pain in joint bones or muscles that lasts seven to ten days**
- **Any fatigue or excessive soreness after a full night's sleep that continues for a number of days**
- **Sharp pain that follows a popping sound**
- **Any unusual or severe pain**
- **Soreness or pain that occurs in the same location every time you run or walk**

DO EFFECTIVE STRETCHING

Describing the importance of stretching, Bob Anderson, the author of *Stretching,* says simply that it relaxes your mind and tunes up your body. And there is no question that proper stretching is an important component of any fitness routine. Stretching helps keep muscles supple, strong, and balanced, so that one muscle group is not overstressed because another is too tight. It promotes flexibility and helps prevent injuries.

If you haven't done much regular exercise before starting your running or walking program, stretching provides an important transition for your muscles and joints. It eases the way toward your more active lifestyle. Stretching is particularly important for runners, since running increases tightness and inflexibility.

During the running boom that began in the late 1960s and early 1970s, conventional wisdom told you to stretch both before and after you ran. Today, thinking on the subject has changed. As described in the section "Begin Gradually," ease into your running and walking and then save your stretching until after your workout, when your muscles are warmed up. You'll obtain more benefits from stretching then and avoid injuries that can occur if you stretch cold, tight muscles and joints.

Stretches should be relaxing, slow movements that gently develop and lengthen your muscles and promote flexibility in your joints. Generally, ease into a stretch as you exhale, hold the stretch for thirty to forty seconds without bouncing, and then repeat. Breathe normally while you stretch. You goal is to feel a pleasant tension during the stretch but not to feel any pain. Please, forget the old image of a woman, bent over at the waist, bouncing to touch her toes. See Chapter 1 for stretching routines that are useful after you run or walk.

A personal note:

> I find the most important stretch I do is after I run. When I finish a really long, hard run, I feel everything has been pounded down. One thing I love to do is reach up and hang from a bar or tree branch and just let my spine straighten out. It really helps.

BEWARE OF THE PERILS OF OVERENTHUSIASM

Although we are familiar with the problem of not keeping up with an exercise program once you start, being too enthusiastic also has its pitfalls. One of the most common causes of preventable injuries is doing too much too soon. You get enthusiastic about your program and don't want to quit or cop out on workouts even if you are feeling a little pain or discomfort that just doesn't go away. You rationalize that it's only a small thing and you can run or walk through it. Perhaps the 5K you've been training for is coming up the next weekend and you don't want to miss it. Please refer to "Listen to Your Body," above. It is telling you something that you can't ignore.

Taking care of small aches and pains may mean missing a few days of workouts. But when the alternative is a larger problem that could cause you to miss significant time, there really isn't any choice. Besides, time away from running or walking doesn't mean time away from all exercise. Explore alternatives such as stationary cycling or swimming so you can continue to work on your fitness. You'll come back to running or walking even stronger than before.

FIND A RUNNING OR WALKING SURFACE
THAT IS KIND TO YOUR BODY

Carefully choose the surface on which you will run or walk. The longer you are on your feet, the kinder the surface should be. Your shoes will absorb road shock, but you can make things even more comfortable if you find a forgiving surface for your workouts.

The hardest surface is concrete, probably the most easily accessible for most of us. However, it is totally unforgiving. Asphalt is a better choice because it is comparatively resilient. If you switch from one to the other, you'll feel the difference immediately. Hard-packed dirt is fabulous, as are mountain or forest trails with hard-packed dirt or pine needles. The Rails to Trails Conservancy is a nationwide organization that is converting unused railroad track beds into excellent running, walking, and biking trails. Call them at 202-331-9696 to find out about trails in your area.

Beach running or walking can be pleasant for most women, except those with tight Achilles tendons, generally women who have worn high heels most of their lives. The soft sand puts a strain on the

Achilles tendon because your heel dips down into the surface, placing a strong stretch on the area that could aggravate any soreness you already have. If you have this problem, hold off your beach running or walking until you have sufficiently stretched out your Achilles tendons. And try to stay down near the shoreline where the sand is firmer and less angled. Some beaches are not flat enough to run on.

If you usually run or walk on roads, be sure to find some flat space every once in a while to compensate for the slight angle you may be training on. Roads are built slightly higher in the center, so the sides are not truly flat surfaces.

KEEP NOTES ON YOUR ACHES AND PAINS

Your running or walking diary can be a terrific resource in preventing injuries. In addition to noting your distances, times, etc., add a few words about small aches and pains, if you have any, or any changes in your routine. If an injury develops, the diary can provide clues to what you were doing as it happened. Did you alter your training program, start to work out on a new surface, or change shoes? Small differences that you may not think are important, or even remember, may emerge as a pattern you can learn from—and not repeat.

BE AWARE OF YOUR TECHNIQUE

A patient of Dr. Miller's, who recently began following a walking program, complained to him about low-back pain. During his examination, he watched her walk and noted she was leaning very far forward with each stride, the likely source of the imbalance that led to the back pain.

Problems of this type can develop if you try to exaggerate your normal walking stride—overstride or develop other distorted walking techniques—when you are fitness walking. The best advice is to use your natural walking pattern.

Think about your form so you don't develop bad habits. Review it in a mirror or ask your running or walking partner, or someone you've gotten to know along your route, to take a look at how your are moving and give you feedback about your technique.

Use mental imaging to keep your technique on target. While running or walking, keep a picture of yourself with perfect form in your mind and strive to achieve that image.

GET ENOUGH SLEEP AND DON'T RUN OR WALK IF YOU'RE FATIGUED

One of the benefits of you'll get from your running or walking program is greater energy. But feeling stronger, more energetic, and in control of yourself doesn't mean you're superwoman. You still need to get enough sleep to keep up the full schedule you're following. Without sufficient rest your body will break down at its weakest point, and that may be a knee or an Achilles tendon that has been giving you some trouble.

By the time we're forty, most of us know all about sleep deprivation. We may even know how much sleep we need to perform at our best. Sleep is an important part of your training routine. It is the time when your body rebuilds muscles that have been pushed and stressed during training. Adequate rest and recovery time make your muscles stronger. The training technique of alternating hard and easy workouts succeeds because of this principle. Without a proper amount of sleep, you'll notice that you are not only tired but your muscles are more likely to be sore and aching. So get your beauty—and exercise—rest.

If you are feeling tired during a workout, don't force yourself to do a preset mileage or time. Injuries often happen at the end of a long run or walk. Fatigue dulls your awareness, and if you're not paying attention, even picking up one foot after the other can become difficult. So don't be afraid to stop when you get tired. There is always tomorrow.

As I mentioned, you need to alternate hard days of running and walking with easy ones. It's also a good idea to take a complete day off every week. Your body needs time to recover and rebuild from the additional effort, just as it does when you are weight training. Recovery days are essential to preventing injuries and allowing your body to progress. You don't have to be inactive on recovery days. Do exercises that use different muscles, like swimming or riding a bike. It is the repeated strain on the same muscles and joints that can cause problems.

RUN OR WALK ON FAMILIAR PATHS, ESPECIALLY EARLY IN THE MORNING AND AT NIGHT

If your schedule forces you to run or walk when it is dark—very early in the morning or at night—make sure to choose a path that has good lighting and that you are familiar with. If you can't see a crack in the pavement or curb, you can't avoid it. Check out your route in advance and make sure there will be sufficient illumination. This applies not only to your health but also your safety.

The Pre-Exercise Physical: What You Need to Find Out and What to Expect

Get a complete physical exam before you start an exercise program: It is probably the most often repeated advice you receive. With the growth and recognition of sports medicine as a medical specialty, the scope of what an exam can accomplish has changed, with important ramifications for injury awareness and prevention.

Beyond the basic physical, your doctor can do an in-depth evaluation of your muscular and skeletal systems to identify risk factors that make you prone to certain injuries. We all have a unique physical makeup with particular strengths and weakness—muscular imbalances, joint instability, congenital or pre-existing conditions, and biomechanical problems—such as the normal tendency for one leg to be longer than the other, which can cause an imbalance in your stride when you walk or run. Proper preventive measures—such as orthodics in your shoes to correct imbalances—are often available, so that these conditions need not necessarily interfere with your exercise plans.

If you have had joint replacement surgery or have a pacemaker, this is the time to check out your exercise plans with your doctor. You and your doctor can work out a plan on what steps you need to take to minimize your risk factors. Then you can start with the confidence that you've chosen the proper exercise for you.

Who would be the best physician to do this type of examination? The answer is varied, but you can start by looking for a doctor who has specialized training in sports medicine and is comfortable working with athletes and people who exercise regularly. A doctor who is familiar with the demands of running and walking would be equipped to advise you on the risks and patterns of injury, as well as how to avoid them.

Ask friends, family, or coworkers who run or walk for recommendations. You can contact your local high school for the name of the physician who examines athletes for their yearly physical. Sometimes local running or walking clubs have a list of preferred doctors in the area. Or you may call on a local doctor who you know is a runner or walker.

Injury Q and A

WHAT SHOULD I DO IF I SUSTAIN AN INJURY?

The first line of defense is a system athletes have come to know as RICE: rest, ice, compression, elevation. Get off your feet and keep the injured area elevated above hip level while you apply ice. You can simply put ice cubes in a plastic bag and wrap it on your injury with a bandage or a towel. My choice is Erogmed, an ice pack you keep in the freezer and that comes with a Velcro closing band to wrap around the injured area; it is secure and eliminates dripping. A package of frozen peas held in place with an Ace bandage is an excellent low-tech alternative.

Applying ice to sore areas works wonders. Not only does the ice soothe an injury and reduce swelling, once it's removed blood rushes into the area to flush out toxins and promote healing with fresh, oxygenated blood.

TIP

Don't put ice directly on bare skin and/or apply it for more than ten minutes at a time.

Some doctors recommend adding another letter to the RICE acronym: P for protect. For instance, if you twisted an ankle, you would leave on your shoe to protect and immobilize the area, then follow the rest of the steps.

If pain persists after following these steps, seek medical attention. Although you are probably doing much of what the doctor will recommend, you should make sure that you don't have a more serious problem that requires additional treatment. Charts at the end of this chapter describe some common injuries, their cause, and treatments.

A personal note:

Sometimes, after a run, I put ice on my Achilles tendons even when they don't hurt, as a preventive measure. I've noticed that I run better the next day, too!

DOES MASSAGE HELP WITH ACHES AND PAINS? DO I NEED TO GO TO A HEALTH CLUB TO GET A MASSAGE?

Getting a massage is an excellent form of treatment. It would be wonderful if we could all afford it regularly. If you have the time and money, do it. It is not a foolish indulgence; professional athletes get massages as a regular part of their training.

A massage relaxes tight muscles; it forces blood into poor circulation areas that are injury-prone, such as the Achilles tendon; and it helps move out accumulations of acids and toxins that are the residue of work and stress.

If you don't have the time or money for a regular massage, you can do it effectively for yourself. Have you ever rubbed your head and neck when you have a headache? It relieves the pain and tension. That's self-massage. After a run or walk, rub areas that take a particular pounding—the bottoms of your feet, Achilles tendon, thighs, and calf muscles. You'll feel better for it. However, if these areas are inflamed or injured, massage gently and moderately until they are healed.

WHAT TYPE OF DOCTORS CAN HELP ME WITH RUNNING OR WALKING INJURIES? WHAT SHOULD I EXPECT FROM THE DOCTOR-PATIENT RELATIONSHIP?

Your family physician, internist, or orthopedist would be a good choice, particularly if he or she has an interest or specialization in sports medicine. Podiatrists and chiropractors are also an excellent option because of their knowledge of foot, muscle, and joint problems so common to runners and walkers.

Look for a doctor who will encourage you to be an active participant in making decisions about your health care. After all, you are taking charge of your health by running or walking and making other lifestyle changes. Your doctor should support you in this effort.

Ideally, you'd like to work with a physician who listens to you, asks you questions, and sees himself or herself as an educator who will help you make the best choices in dealing with injuries or other health-related questions. If your doctor doesn't want to bring you into the process of taking care of your health, then you may want to find one who does.

WHAT IF I HAVE PRE-EXISTING PROBLEMS, WITH MY KNEES OR BACK FOR EXAMPLE? WOULD THAT RULE OUT RUNNING OR WALKING?

Not necessarily, although it maybe a factor in deciding which exercise you choose to pursue. The pre-exercise physical would be the time to discuss these issues with your doctor and find out what you can do lessen the impact these conditions may have on your exercise and vice versa. For instance, you may need to do additional stretches or use an orthotic device in your shoes. Indeed, regular exercise may help alleviate some the physical problems you are suffering with.

Low-back pain affects nearly 80 percent of people at one point or another and, most often, it is not caused by running. However, it is a problem that can be helped by preventive measures such as exercises to strengthen the abdominal muscles and proper stretching after running or walking.

HOW DO YOU COME BACK AFTER AN INJURY?

Resume your running or walking schedules very gradually after an injury. Most reinjuries occur within a few months after you've resumed exercising, because you're overanxious and do too much too quickly If you have been able to do alternative forms of exercise, your fitness level may be very good, but don't push yourself too fast. Use the charts in chapters 3 and 4 to reestablish your training program. You may have to go back a bit at first, but if you're careful you'll get back to your previous level—maybe even beyond it.

WHAT ABOUT SURGERY TO REPAIR AN INJURY?

If you have a serious injury, you may eventually require surgery to repair it. But surgery should be a last resort. Try alternative methods of handling the injury, then get *three* medical opinions before you commit to surgery. Taking time off completely can often do wonders.

I'VE HEARD SO MUCH ABOUT BONE LOSS, OSTEOPOROSIS, AND EXERCISE. CAN I EXERCISE BEFORE AND AFTER MENOPAUSE WITHOUT RISKING BONE FRACTURES?

These are complicated issues for which there is no single formula or answer. You will need to look at your medical history, lifestyle, heredity, and other risk factors in terms of bone loss or your likelihood to have osteoporosis.

Bones are not static. They are growing and renewing themselves throughout our lives, although bone density loss probably begins in our thirties. As you get older, new bone forms more slowly, and the body's ability to absorb calcium diminishes. Weight-bearing exercises such as running or fitness walking combined with proper calcium intake will help maintain bone strength and density. So if you are over forty and not menopausal, exercise is recommended as part over an overall approach to bone mass retention.

Once you reach menopause, there is a rapid decline in bone mass. The best treatment to reduce the severity of this loss is a combination of estrogen replacement therapy, sufficient intake of calcium (1,200–1,500 milligrams per day is recommended), and exercise, such as running or brisk walking. Doctors believe this multifaceted approach is most valuable in slowing bone loss. Exercising and calcium alone are not generally thought to be sufficient. Since the lack of estrogen is a key factor in the loss of bone mass, some form of hormone replacement should be considered. However, you should make a decision about estrogen replacement therapy or its alternatives separately from your choice of exercise.

One other factor in bone mass deterioration is the effect of a sedentary lifestyle. Lack of physical activity also contributes to a loss of bone density. If you have been active all of your life and suddenly stop exercising, you'll experience a reduction in bone mass. Similarly, if you're not active after menopause, your bone mass loss can be more severe. And while lifelong exercise would be ideal, anytime you start to exercise you can begin to receive benefits, such as slowing post-menopause bone mass loss.

Osteoporosis is a specific illness in which the loss of bone mass and deterioration in bone structure make bones extremely fragile and vulnerable to fracturing as a result of falls or even normal, everyday activities. There are numerous risk factors for osteoporosis (see Chapter 10), and you need to have a bone density test to determine if you have the condition. Although it has not been shown that exercise prevents osteoporosis, most doctors who have studied the disease believe that older women should participate in activities that will improve their strength, flexibility, balance, and coordination to lessen their vulnerability to falling and the subsequent fractures that are so common to the disease.

I'VE ALWAYS WORN HIGH HEELS. DO I NEED TO DO ANY SPECIAL PREPARATION WHEN I START MY RUNNING OR WALKING PROGRAM?

Dr. Lori Weisenfeld, a New York City podiatrist, says that women who have worn high heels for decades often have difficulty adjusting to flat shoes like running or walking sneakers. "From all those years of wearing high heels, their Achilles tendon, which is in the back of the leg just above the ankle, becomes very tight. Running and walking shoes will stretch the tendon and cause pain in the calves and up to the back." In order to avoid this problem, Dr. Weisenfeld says it's important to do stretches specifically for your calf and hamstring muscles. Since it will take some time to achieve the flexibility you need, she recommends adding heel lifts to your athletic shoes, which you can remove once the Achilles tendons are more flexible.

IF I HAD KNEE OR HIP REPLACEMENT SURGERY, WHAT KIND OF EXERCISE SHOULD I BE DOING?

Exercise is an important part of the long-term recovery process after joint replacement surgery. Doctors recommend moderate, weight-bearing exercise such as walking, running, treadmill walking, and doubles tennis. They also suggest a weight-training program. Water aerobics and bike riding, although not weight bearing, are good complementary exercises. Exercise will build up your muscle strength, help you control your weight, and promote flexibility and balance—all benefits to your future health after this type of surgery. Work with your doctor to create the exercise program that is best for you.

FOOT INJURY CHART

(Although some of these injuries are on the leg, their origin is in the foot.)

Injury	Symptoms	Causes	Treatment
Anterior shin splints	Throbbing pain on the front and outer side of shinbone.	Usually found in high-arch foot or supinator. More common in walkers than runners because they use anterior muscles more. Often occurs when you walk or run on hills or wear shoes that are too wide or loose. Tight calf muscles.	Slow pace. Check shoes for extreme wear. Strengthen muscle by standing or sitting with heel firmly on the ground and tapping the ball of your foot until the muscle gets fatigued. Repeat with other foot. Stretch calf muscles by pointing toe to floor. Ice area.
Blisters	Painful fluid-filled sacs under the skin	Friction: against too-tight shoes, wrinkled sock, or hot road surface.	Cleanse area with anti-septic. With sterilized needle, pierce blister at base. Gently squeeze out fluid. Coat blister and opening with Neosporin. Cover lightly. Try not to irritate the area. If you must run or walk on it, cover with second skin and continue to treat with Neosporin.

Injury	Symptoms	Causes	Treatment
Posterior shin splints	Pain and throbbing sensation on inner part of the shin. Diffused pain up and down inner part of leg.	If arch is collapsing, the muscle attached to the shin that supports the arch can be overworked. Pronation or flat arches. Training on hard surfaces. Over-training or too rapid increase in training.	Rest. Apply ice and take and anti-inflammatory medication. Slow training program. Try a more supportive shoe. Consider wearing orthotics, over-the-counter or custom-made arch supports.
Black toenail syndrome	Blood collects under toenail, turning it black.	Shoes are too short so ends of toes jam against the front of the shoe. Shoes are too large, causing a lot of foot motion with toes bumping against the front of the shoe.	Keep toenails cut short. Buy correct size shoes. May require nail to be opened to relieve pressure.
Plantar fasciatis	Pulling, tearing sensation in the arch or heel. Feels as if you stepped on a stone and bruised your heel. Usually feels worse when you wake up in the morning.	Excessive pronation or high arches. When arch collapses during exercise, fascia becomes tight and pulls.	Rest. Wear a support rather than a cushioning shoe. Do calf stretches. Get heel lifts or get fitted for orthotics.
Fallen or dropped arches	Pain in arches.	Overuse injury. Can be an inherited tendency. Overweight.	Cut back on workouts. Toe curl exercises to strengthen the arches.

Injury	Symptoms	Causes	Treatment
Sesamoiditis	Pain on the bottom of big toe joint.	Bruise to the sesamoid bones, two small bones under the ball of the foot. Often caused by uphill or downhill running or walking.	Cushion area by placing a small pad right behind the bones. Pad can be worn in both regular and athletic shoes.
Bunions and hammertoes	Pressure and pain on bunion. Develop corns or blisters.	Pressure created on bunion because of incorrect shoe.	Purchase a shoe that accommodates bunions and hammertoes without causing pressure. Orthotics. Consider surgery as a last resort.
Corns and calluses	Pain on bottom of the foot or between toes. Corns are circular in shape and occur at a pressure point. Callus is a more diffuse area of thickened skin.	Corns are caused by pressure. Calluses result from friction.	Purchase properly fitted shoe. Corn pads can help cushion area. A pumice stone can remove excess skin. If they are too large or thick, see a podiatrist to have both removed.
Knee pain	Pain and inflammation behind kneecap after exercise.	Women have a wider pelvis than men and that may result in a a crossover in their running or walking stride that stresses knee. Incorrect tracking of the kneecap due to lack of thigh muscle strength. Can also be caused by overpronation.	Select a shoe that controls overpronation. Exercises to strengthen quadriceps (thigh muscles) that can hold knee in proper track. Ice knees. Over-the-counter or prescription orthotics.

Orthotics can make a big difference in your running or walking. They correct imbalances in your biomechanics. Many, many top runners must wear orthotics because they run so many miles that normal body imbalances become exaggerated. For you, orthotics can make the difference between running or walking pain-free or not exercising at all. A pre-exercise visit with a podiatrist to see if you can benefit from orthotics can prevent a lot of discomfort later on. Once you have orthotics, check them for wear and "flattening out" just as you do your running or walking shoes.

LEG AND BACK INJURY CHART

Injury	Symptoms	Causes	Treatment
Calf muscle strains	Sudden pain and possible swelling in calf muscle.	Overtraining, lack of flexibility, improper warm-up, incorrect footgear. Dehydration.	Ice, rest, physical therapy or deep massage. Drink a lot of water. Limit wieght-bearing activities. Stretching and light restrengthening once area is pain free.
Hamstring muscles	Chronic, sometimes spastic, throbbing pain anywhere along the muscle from the lower buttock to behind the knee.	Overuse, excessive speed training, poor warm-up, inflexibility, or running when injured. Imbalance between hamstring and quadricep strength. One leg shorter than the other.	RICE. Slow, short runs; deep massage; judicious use of anti-inflammatory drugs; strengthening program for quadriceps, if an examination determines they are weak. Light stretching of hamstring.

Injury	Symptoms	Causes	Treatment
Stress fracture	Pinpoint pain in bone. Present on weight bearing (e.g., getting out of bed in the morning). Pain starts suddenly. Need bone scan, CT, or X ray for definite diagnosis.	Overtraining, rapid increase in training, overpronation or flat arches, hard or hilly training surfaces. Running or walking on crowned surfaces. Leg length inequalities.	Total rest from any weight-bearing activity for six to eight weeks. May need hand crutches. You can continue to work out with such activities as pool training, stationary bicycling, and swimming. Have leg lengths assessed; consider shoe lift to normalize.
Groin muscles and stress fractures	Sharp pain while running or walking in groin muscles, either from the inside of the leg down to the knee or from the pelvis up to upper part of the the groin. Stress fracture: severe pain that increases with standing. Requires bone scan to diagnose.	Usually caused by overuse—excessively long runs or speed work. Can also result from slipping on ice or upward curve of a road	Rest away from running and walking.
Low-back pain	Strain in lower-back muscles or that extends to buttock or lower leg.	Most back pain is not running related. However, continuing to run or walk if you have severe back pain can aggravate the condition.	Temporary rest, physical therapy, prescriptive exercises, including easy walking. Keep back out of drafts. When ready, strengthen abdominal muscles.

Everyone has a some physical idiosyncrasy that can prove troublesome when you run or walk. I've got weird feet. Truly. I inherited bunions and a too-long second toe. My feet look like hell, but they're strong and they work. I can remember when I trained for big marathons that my toenails would fill with blood and I'd have them drilled to relieve the pressure. Sounds gross, but it didn't hurt. Then the toenail would "die" and fall off. The happiest days in my training were when I could run toenail free. Now, I cut out the ends of my shoes when I train long distances. I look like Charlie Chaplin as the "Little Tramp," but my toenails are fine and I don't care.

RESOURCES

Information

Aerobics and Fitness Association of America (AFAA)
15250 Ventura Boulevard
Suite 200
Sherman Oaks, CA 91403
800-233-4886
Membership organization with information about trainers and fitness
    issues.

American Chiropractic Association
1701 Clarendon Boulevard
Arlington, VA 22209
703-276-8800
Membership organization for chiropractic profession.

American College of Sports Medicine
PO Box 1440
Indianapolis, IN 46202
317-637-9200
Information about sports medicine and health topics.

American Dietetic Association
National Center for Nutrition and Dietetics
216 West Jackson Boulevard
Suite 800
Chicago, IL 60606
312-899-0040
800-366-1655 (nutrition hotline)
Provides referrals to sports nutritionists.

American Medical Women's Association
801 North Fairfax Street
Suite 400
Alexandria, VA 22314
703-838-0500
Organization of women doctors that provides information on women's
    health topics.

American Orthopedic Foot and Ankle Society
701 16th Avenue
Seattle, WA 98122
800-235-4855
Information about foot problems.

American Running and Fitness Association
4405 East West Highway
Suite 405
Bethesda, MD 20814
301-913-9517
Membership organization for people interested in running and fitness.

Avon Running—Global Women's Circuit
1345 Avenue of the Americas
26th Floor
New York, NY 10105
212-282-5350
http://www.avon.running.com
Worldwide series of women's 10K runs and 5K walks.

Food and Nutrition Information Center
National Agriculture Library
Beltsville, MD 20705
Answers questions on nutrition.

Melpomene Institute for Women's Health
c/o Judy Mahle Lutter
1010 University Avenue
St. Paul, MN 55104
612 642-1951
Organization dedicated to research about women's health and sports.

National Council on the Aging
409 3rd Street, SW
Washington, DC 20024
800-424-9046

National Master's News
PO Box 16597
North Hollywood, CA 91615
Official publication of World Association of Veteran Athletes and also
    USA Track and Field Association Master's Athletes; page 3 has
    roster of master's running contacts.

National Osteoporosis Foundation
1150 17th Street, NW
Suite 500
Washington, DC 20036
202-223-2226
Provides information about osteoporosis.

National Women's Health Network
1325 G Street, NW
Washington, DC 20005
202-347-1140

National Women's Health Resource Center (NWHRC)
2240 M Street, NW
Suite 201
Washington, DC 20037
202-293-6045

North American Racewalk Foundation
c/o Visha Sedlak
PO Box 18323
Boulder, CO 80308

President's Council on Physical Fitness and Sports
200 Independence Ave., SW
Room 739-H
Washington, DC 20201
202-690-9000

Prevention Walking Club
PO Box 7488
Red Oak, IA 51591
800-666-1216

Road Runners Club of America (RRCA)
1150 South Washington Street
Alexandria, VA 22314
703-836-0558
Association of more than six hundred running clubs; information on
    local running clubs and events.

Southern California Walkers
c/o Elaine Ward
1000 San Pasqual #35
Pasadena, CA 91106

United States Track and Field Association
PO Box 120
Indianapolis, IN 46206
Local associations, contacts, and events.

Walkers Club of America
c/o Howard Jacobson
33 Saddle Lane
Levittown, NY 11756
516-579-WALK

Women's Sports Foundation
Eisenhower Park
East Meadow, NY 11554
800-227-3988
Promotes women's participation in sports.

Books and Videos

NUTRITION

Jane Brody. *Jane Brody's Good Food Book.* New York: Bantam Books, 1987.

Nancy Clark. *Nancy Clark's Sports Nutrition Guidebook.* 2d ed. Champaign, IL: Human Kinetics, 1997.

Nancy Clark. *The New York City Marathon Cookbook.* Nashville: Rutledge Hill Press, 1994.

HEALTH

Boston Women's Health Book Collective. *The New Our Bodies, Ourselves.* New York: Simon & Schuster, 1994.

Jane Brody. *Jane Brody's The New York Times Guide to Personal Health.* New York: Times Books, 1987.

Paul B. Doress-Worters and Diana Laskin Siegal. *The New Ourselves, Growing Older.* New York: Simon & Schuster, 1994.

Naomi Lucks and Melene Smith. *A Women's Midlife Companion.* Rocklin, CA: Prima Publishing, 1997.

Judy Mahle Lutter and Lynn Jafee. *The Bodywise Woman.* Rev. ed. Champaign, IL: Human Kinetics, 1996.

Miriam E. Nelson and Sarah Wernick. *Strong Women Stay Young.* New York: Bantam, 1997.

Mona Shangold and Gabe Mirkin, M.D. *The Complete Sports Medicine Book for Women.* Rev. ed. New York: Simon & Schuster, 1992.

Gail Sheehy. *The Silent Passage.* New York: Pocket Books, 1995.

WALKING

Ron Laird, *The Art of Fast Walking*, Ashtabula: Ron Laird Publishing, 1997.

Howard Jacobson, *Race Walk to Fitness*, New York: Simon & Schuster, 1980.

Marin Rudow, *Maximum Walking*, (video) Seattle: Technique Productions, 1996; 1800-WALK-MAX.

Kathy Smith. *Walkfit for a Better Body.* New York: Warner Books, 1994.

RUNNING

Amby Burfoot, ed. *Runner's World's Complete Book of Running.* Emmaus, PA: Rodale, 1997.

Bob Glover and Shelly-Lynn Florence Glover. *The Runner's Training Diary.* New York: Penguin, 1997.

Annemarie Jutel. *The New Zealand Guide to Women's Running.* Dunedin: Longacre Press, 1995.

Fred Lebow, Gloria Auerbach, and Friends. *The New York Road Runners Club Complete Book of Running.* New York: Random House, 1992.

Roger Robinson. *Heroes and Sparrows.* Auckland: Southwestern Publishing, 1986.

Joan Benoit Samuelson and Gloria Auerbach. *Running for Women.* Emmaus, PA: Rodale, 1995.

Grete Waitz and Gloria Auerbach. *On the Run.* Emmaus, PA: Rodale, 1997.

About the Author

Thirty years ago, an irate official tried forcibly to remove Kathrine Switzer from the 1967 Boston Marathon—simply because she was a woman. Yet Switzer went on to finish the race and become the first woman officially to run the race. Her experiences at that event inspired her to create the innovative Avon International Running Circuit twenty years ago. Now she is back at Avon as program director of the newly re-created Avon Running—Global Women's Circuit series after spending more than a decade in sports broadcasting, sports promotion, and motivational speaking.

From 1977 to 1986, Switzer served as director of Avon Sports Programs and was responsible for the company's worldwide sponsorship of women's running, tennis, and ice-skating events. At its height, the program was active in twenty-one countries, had more than two hundred events, and involved over a million women. In 1986, Switzer formed her own company, Atalanta Sports Promotions, Inc., and embarked on a career in broadcasting and journalism, which has included work for ABC, NBC, CBS, and Turner Sports Broadcasting. She has covered such high-profile events as the Olympic and Goodwill Games, as well as eighteen Boston Marathons, thirteen New York City

Marathons, twelve Pittsburgh Marathons, and six Los Angeles Marathons. In 1997, she won an Emmy Award for her work on the Los Angeles Marathon.

Switzer received both her B.A. and M.A. degrees from Syracuse University's Newhouse School of Journalism. She is a featured columnist in *Marathon & Beyond* and *Women Today*, and her articles have appeared in the *New York Times*, the *Washington Post*, *Runner's World*, and other publications. Switzer, with Avon's support, was a driving force to get the women's marathon event included in the Olympic Games beginning in 1984. She has received numerous citations and awards for her efforts in advancing sports opportunities for women, including a New York State Regents Medal of Excellence, the Billie Jean King Award from the Women's Sports Foundation, Runner of the Decade commendation by *Runner's World* magazine, and an Honor Fellow citation from the National Association of Girls and Women in Sports. Switzer has run thirty-five marathons; she won the 1974 New York City Marathon and competes frequently in age-group running events. She is married to Roger Robinson, Ph.D., professor of English at Victoria University in Wellington, New Zealand, a noted author, commentator, and world-ranked age-group runner.